ELIQ MARANIK

Probiotic Blends
Smoothies and more

INVIGORATING RECIPES
FOR DYNAMIC DIGESTION!

h.f.ullmann

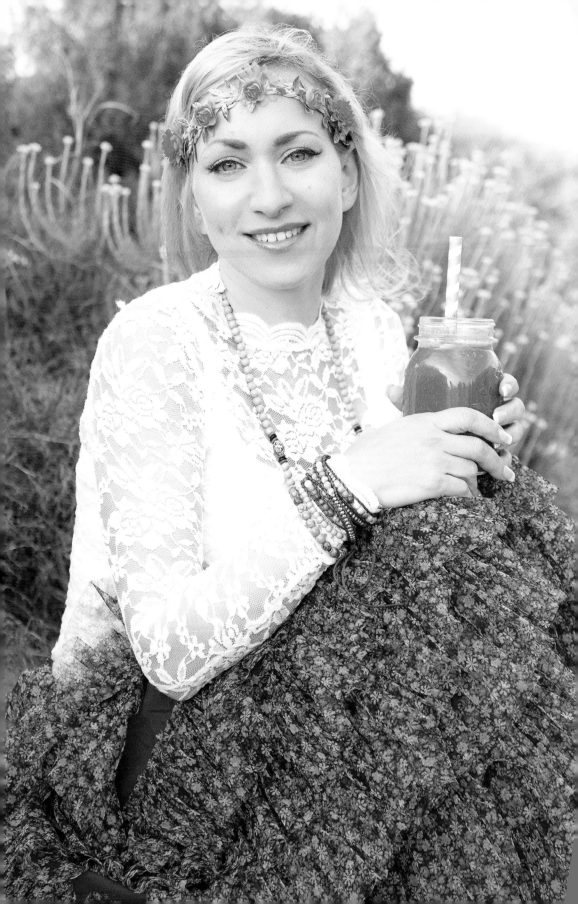

I dedicate this book to my friend Helen, who is at least as crazy as I am about trying out various diets, elixirs, and beneficial and environmentally sustainable habits while never compromising on flavor. Thank you for introducing me to my first SCOBY (a symbiotic culture of bacteria and yeast), for your inspiration, our conversations, your tips and tricks, and, most of all, thank you for your friendship over the past 20 years.

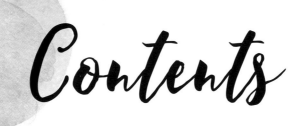

Contents

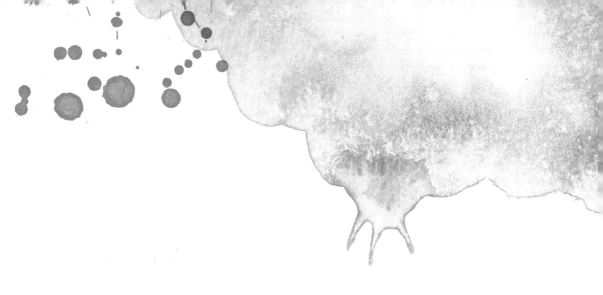

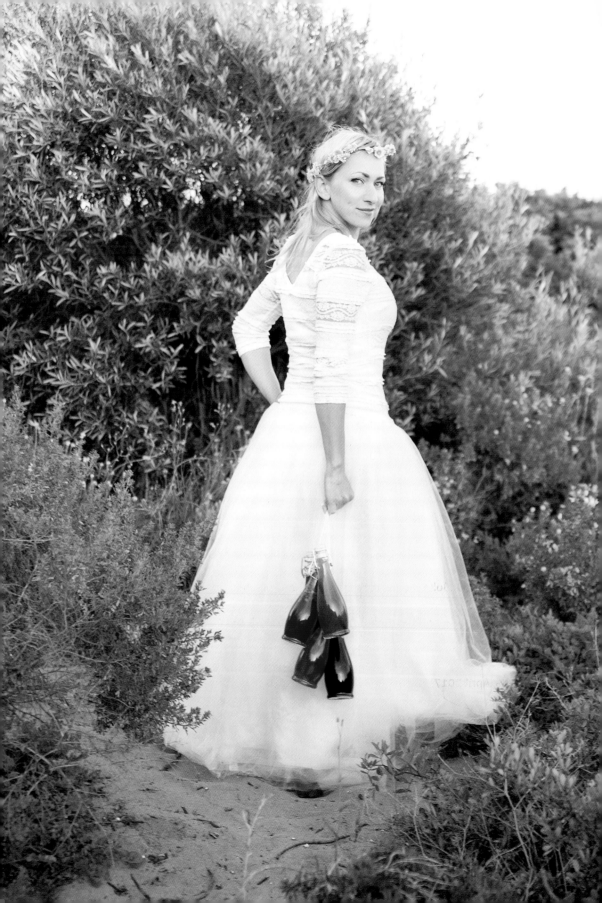

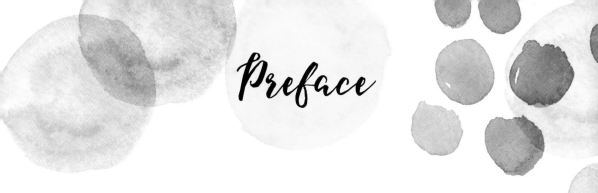

PROBIOTIC SMOOTHIES—A COMBINATION OF BENEFICIAL BACTERIA AND ALL THINGS HEALTHY

A few weeks ago, I attended the launch of the OsteoStrong bone health solution, organized by my friends Gary and Nicholas at their clinic in Marbella, Spain. My first instinct was to decline the invitation, as the deadline for the book you hold in your hands was fast approaching, and I was already running behind. There is something to be gained from every experience, though, and had I never attended this event, I would never have understood my keen interest in probiotics. In the course of the event, I was introduced to a Dr. John Jaquish, a remarkably knowledgeable scientist and doctor from San Francisco, USA. He asked me a question (a fairly obvious one in retrospect) but one that no one had asked me before, one that I had never thought about or, perhaps, one that I had just ignored. The question was: had I taken a lot of antibiotics as a child? I said "No—I'd received them only on a few occasions." However, I was not totally sure, so when the event ended, I called my mom to check. She revealed to me that, from the age of only six months old, I had received antibiotics several times a year for a chronic ear infection and tonsillitis, and that I had refused to have my tonsils removed. Suddenly I realized why I had had stomach cramps my entire life. On the other hand, my tummy troubles forced me to be careful about what I ate and to lead a relatively healthy lifestyle, which I am happy for.

Meeting Dr. Jaquish got me thinking and I found myself remembering things I had forgotten or chosen to forget. At once all the pieces fell into place, and I realized why, from an early age, I had wanted to give everything a try—from annual colonics, all manner of herbs, health preparations, elixirs, and probiotic capsules, to making my own health drinks using kombucha, kefir, and yogurt—all in an attempt to cope with my stomach problems.

I wish to thank Dr. John Jaquish for our exciting conversations and for asking the right questions.

To you, my readers, I wish a life full of many beneficial bacteria.

Eliq Maranik,

Marbella, April 2017

Dr. John Jaquish is the man behind OsteoStrong, a tailored exercise program that strengthens the body and alleviates many types of pain and physical weakness, including osteoporosis: a disease all too common among the elderly. His interest in bone health began with him wanting to help his mom, who herself suffered from osteoporosis. To this very day, Dr Jaquish continues to help thousands of people live healthier lives. Several scientific studies have shown that it is possible to alleviate and even remedy osteoporosis.

To find out more about Dr. John Jaquish, please visit www.johnjaquish.com. For information about OsteoStrong, please visit www.osteostrong.me.

Good gut flora is the key to good health

It has been known for a long time that a well-functioning stomach is essential for good health generally. Hippocrates declared that all illness begins in the gut, and the more we find out, the more we realize how right he was.

PROBIOTICS—YOUR GUT'S BEST FRIEND

Beneficial gut bacteria live in symbiosis with humans, preventing and relieving illness. Each person's gastrointestinal system contains around 100,000 billion bacteria of various types, all carrying out numerous important functions day and night. Another term for these good bacteria is probiotics, sometimes called "the gut's best friend".

Gut flora and a healthy stomach are crucial in enabling us to get the benefit of the food we eat. A healthy gut with a healthy bacterial culture has the ability to break down our food and increase the take-up of nutrients. The production of B and K vitamins is also dependent on proper gut function. The bacteria in your small intestine can produce a certain amount of B12, while the bacteria in the large intestine can produce vitamins K, B1, B2, B6, and B9. A healthy stomach makes for a healthy person!

The good bacteria also help to strengthen the immune system, reduce the risk of allergies, combat IBS and stomach ulcers, prevent vaginal yeast infections, reduce the side effects of antibiotics, and also counteract common, everyday stomach problems such as diarrhea, bloating, and stomach ache. There is also much to suggest that mental health is improved if the stomach is working as it should.

PREBIOTICS

Prebiotics is the collective term for a type of carbohydrate that the body absorbs slowly and fibers that are non-digestible. These include oligosaccharides, which stimulate the growth of healthy gut bacteria—probiotics. Prebiotics also have a beneficial effect on the pH of the gut, increase the take-up of essential minerals, and combat the negative effects of sugar. Prebiotics are found naturally in items such as pulses, milk, onions, tomatoes, bananas, oats, garlic, and honey. For best results, prebiotics and probiotics should be balanced.

HOW DID OUR ANCESTORS LIVE?

People have always eaten food that promotes the growth of probiotic bacteria, but the way we live today is dramatically different from the life our forefathers led. These days, we eat a lot of fast food and are under constant stress, and so it is not surprising that our gut flora gets out of balance, so giving the harmful bacteria an opportunity to develop.

Fermented foods have always been part of the human diet. Eating such foods is a natural, simple way to make sure you get the good bacteria needed to keep your stomach working properly. The consumption of the type of food that produces beneficial bacteria fell dramatically once fridges started appearing in people's homes, as there was less need to ferment food to keep it fresh.

I try to live as my ancestors did as far as possible, which means I eat food that is pure, additive-free, and not produced by chemical means. I prefer naturally fermented or lacto-fermented foods, which are a fantastic source of both prebiotics and probiotic, good bacteria.

BACTERIA CULTURES WITH A HISTORY

We humans have not always known how certain foods help to promote a well-functioning stomach and good health, but our ancestors noticed that they made a difference and ate them to keep themselves healthy. Kombucha tea is a Chinese health drink that has been made for many thousands of years. Asian cultures have long eaten soy sauce, miso soup, and lacto-fermented vegetables such as kimchi. The ancient Romans regularly ate fermented cabbage, just as the Germans do. In India, *lassi*, a yogurt drink, is consumed before a meal. In Eastern Europe and Russia, *kefir* has been part of the diet as long as anyone can remember, and the *yogurt* of Greece and Turkey has a long history.

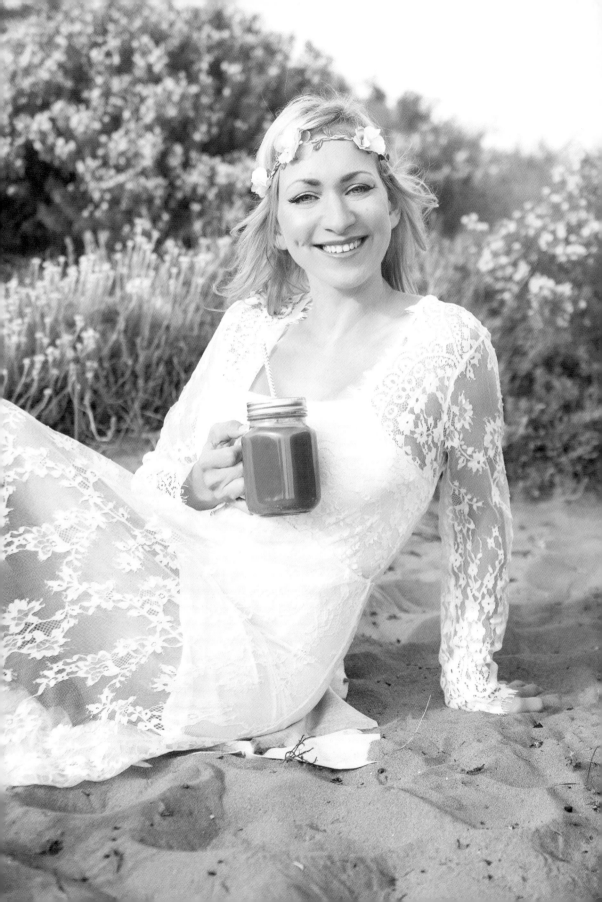

HUMANS ARE 90 PERCENT BACTERIA

Our gut is home to countless bacteria, some good, some bad. The walls of the large intestine contain several pounds of bacteria and are covered with 100,000 billion bacteria of something between 300 and 1,000 different varieties. Our ancestors could have up to 2,500 different varieties of bacteria out of the 6,500 that have been identified. There are ten times as many bacteria as the total number of cells in the body. Maintaining the ideal balance between good and bad bacteria is key to good physical and mental health.

Our world is one of chemical controls, preservatives, food additives, overuse of antibiotics, and stress. Because of this, the bacteria that are essential to good gut flora are becoming scarcer. We should have 80 percent good gut bacteria and 20 percent bad bacteria, but because of poor diet and acid-forming foods, many people today have only 20 percent of the good bacteria and 80 percent of the bad bacteria.

PROBIOTICS—TABLETS, POWDER, AND CAPSULES

There has been an increasing interest in supplementary probiotics in recent years, but the majority of all probiotics sold, either in tablet, powder, or capsule form, are synthetic and some are even genetically modified. Similarly, most do not contain any prebiotics—the nourishment that keep our gut flora in good shape and promotes the growth of probiotics. So select your capsules carefully and try different makes. Different brands contain different bacteria, so find the one that suits you best, and ring the changes. Your gut has hundreds of different types of bacteria, and if you make sure that you take in a good variety you are more likely to be successful in topping up the bacteria that are in short supply. So preparations that contain ten different types of bacteria are better than a preparation that only contains one. For mild stomach problems, or for preventive purposes, you might need a supplement of 1–2 billion bacteria each day. In more serious cases, 25–100 billion bacteria per day might be necessary, particularly after treatment with antibiotics. But always start modestly and increase intake accordingly.

STORE-BOUGHT FERMENTED PRODUCTS

If you do not have time to make your own fermented food and drink, there are good options in the stores, and more and more are coming on stream all the time. Increasing numbers of us are now becoming aware of the importance of these foods for gut flora and health in general. Examples of such products are kefir, kombucha, yogurt, fermented dairy products, sauerkraut, kimchi, pickled and fermented vegetables, soy sauce, and miso soup. But be sure to read the packaging: drinks and fermented dishes should be fermented by means of a natural fermentation process and must on no account be pasteurized. All too often, vinegar is used instead of fermentation, and even if a natural fermentation process has been used, the product may have been heated so that it becomes germ-free—that means it has none of the probiotic bacteria left.

TREATMENT WITH ANTIBIOTICS

If you are starting a course of antibiotics, always start taking probiotics at the same time—do not wait until after you have finished treatment. Sometimes it is absolutely essential to take antibiotics, and you really have no choice. Most people know that antibiotics have a detrimental effect on gut flora because they kill many probiotic bacteria, which can have long-term consequences for health—fungal overgrowth is one of them.

The walls of the large intestine contain several pounds of bacteria and are covered with about 100,000 billion bacteria of something between 300 and 1,000 different varieties. Our ancestors could have up to 2,500 different varieties of bacteria out of the 6,500 that have been identified.

STERILE AT BIRTH

While it is in its mother's womb, a child is completely sterile and essentially free of bacteria. But the moment it passes through the birth canal it is exposed to its mother's bacteria, which rapidly colonize. A child born by Caesarean section is exposed to different bacteria, and this can have negative consequences. Breastfeeding is also important for ensuring that a child acquires lots of good bacteria. Studies of children that have not been breastfed have noted a connection between a higher instance of allergies and a lower level of variation in gut bacteria.

DO GUT BACTERIA MAKE YOU FAT?

It has been observed that certain bacteria can affect how much fat is taken up and stored by the body. They also seem to be able to influence your appetite, what food you fancy, and thus the sort of food you actually eat. So two people who want to lose weight, eat exactly the same food, and do the same amount of exercise can have different outcomes. There might be several factors in the body at play, but it does depend partly on the bacteria. So, gut bacteria can contribute to weight increase.

WHAT CAUSES THE FARTING?

We all produce on average two liters of intestinal gas each day. When our gut bacteria get to work on the residue of our food so that it starts to ferment, various gases are formed, including carbon dioxide, hydrogen, methane, or the infamous hydrogen sulfide that smells of rotten eggs. Those who have problems with over-frequent or excessively odorous farts often have an imbalance in their gut bacteria and/or poor digestion.

THE GUT FUNCTIONS AS A SECOND BRAIN

The gut produces more serotonin—a feel-good hormone that enhances your mood—than the brain. So what is responsible for making you feel low? Is it your brain or your gut bacteria? What determines your mood and how you feel? If you feel down, worried, or depressed for no apparent reason, it may be due to problems in your gut...

TOP UP WITH GOOD BACTERIA EVERY DAY

The challenge is to find a way of balancing the good flora by introducing probiotics so that the digestive system can function at its best.

You can do this in two ways:
- ♥ probiotic and fermented food
- ♥ probiotic dietary supplements

I normally have one natural, fermented drink a day. If I am traveling, I take probiotic capsules.

MY TROUBLESOME TUMMY

The effect that your gut flora has on your health cannot be stressed enough. An imbalance in your gut bacteria can often result in serious problems, and many illnesses, both physical and mental, are said to stem from the digestive system.

Having lived most of my life with a troublesome tummy, I have tried most things, and I find that home-made probiotics work better than anything else I have tested—provided I vary them and take them regularly. When I started working to achieve balance in my stomach, I found there were other positive effects such as increased energy, an improvement in my mood, better sleep, and a healthy loss of weight.

Having spent hundreds of hours of reading, testing, and brewing, I have learned how to produce my probiotic drinks myself. They are cheap, simple to make, and also quite delicious. I have written this book to share everything I have learned through testing and tasting.

For positive results, all you need to do is to remember to eat probiotics regularly and to alternate between different products, such as kefir, kombucha, rejuvelac, yogurt, fermented vegetables, and sauerkraut.

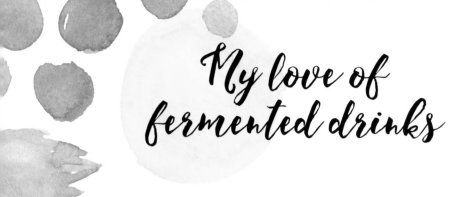

My love of fermented drinks

I am a great fan of fermented drinks, and I love making them myself from scratch. My grandmother and her friends often gave me fermented drinks when I was a child, and perhaps that was what aroused my interest in healthy lifestyles. Of course, I have also been influenced by my travels throughout the world, including visits to the amazing health bars of New York and Florida.

Fermented drinks are carbonated and thus have a similarity with soft drinks. Maybe the huge success of the soft drinks industry is due to our bodies having some residual memory of a drink that is essential for health and survival. But of course soft drinks are anything but healthy, and definitely do not contain any probiotics. I hope that this book will inspire all my readers to try out new, simply delicious drinks brimming with vitamins, minerals, antioxidants, and probiotics.

I do have three favorites:

♥ **KOMBUCHA**, the first fermented drink I made for myself. I still love it more and more every day. I flavor it in a thousand different ways, and now my three-year-old daughter loves it too.

♥ **KEFIR**, my grandmother's neighbor taught me to make this as a child.

♥ **REJUVELAC**, which I learned to make after reading Ann Wigmore's fantastic book about wheatgrass and how she could use it to cure most illnesses.

NB:
The different cultures must be kept at least a meter apart, otherwise bacteria might accidentally be split between different glass jars which could weaken the cultures.

You can keep several cultures going simultaneously, e.g., kombucha, kefir, rejuvelac, sourdough, etc., but note that *the different cultures must be kept at least a meter apart*, otherwise bacteria might accidently be split between different glass jars which could weaken the cultures.

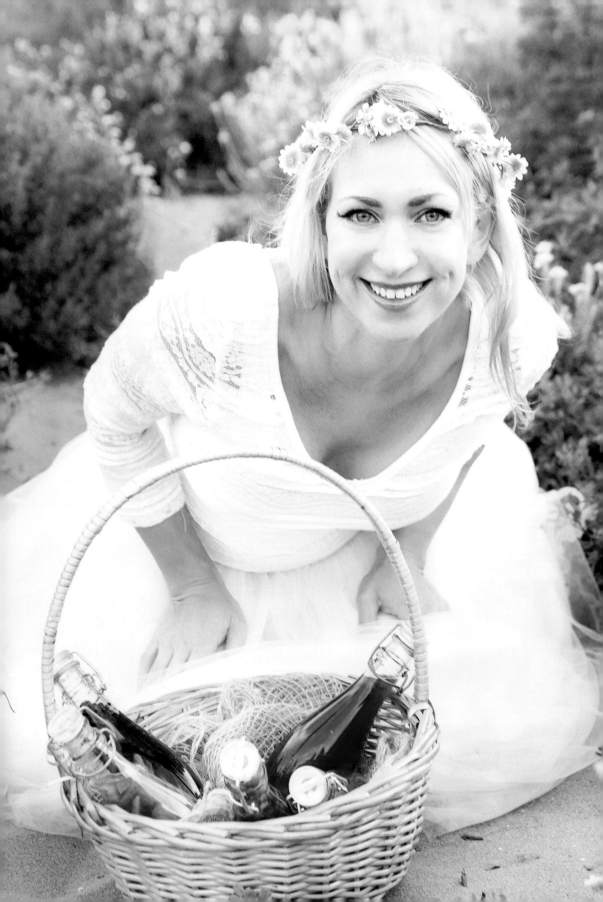

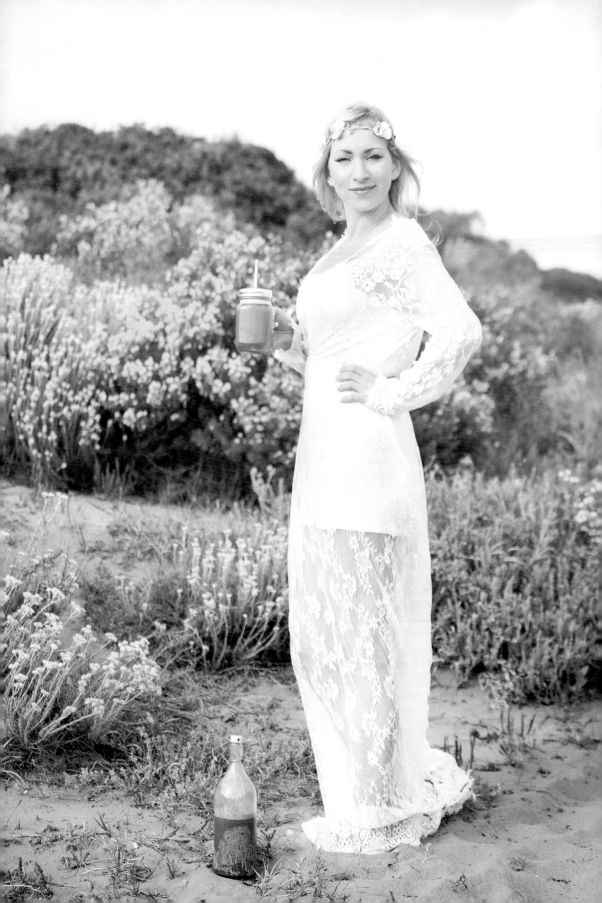

Kombucha

In ancient, traditional Chinese medicine, kombucha tea is considered to be the drink of immortality and the elixir of life. It was being drunk as early as 200 BC and, according to its advocates, has many health-promoting properties, including benefits to digestion and complexion, and reduced body and joint pain. Like other probiotic drinks, kombucha keeps hunger pangs at bay and eases problems in the gut, such as gas, constipation, and the side effects of antibiotics and other medical treatment. It also boosts the immune system, preventing colds and flu. Nutrients in kombucha include lactic bacteria, acetic acid, polysaccharides, vitamins C, E, K, B1, B2, B3, B6, and B12, and a range of minerals—iron, sodium, manganese, magnesium, potassium, copper, and zinc.

I am so in love with kombucha—it is my absolute favorite, super-duper health drink. I drink it every day, and every day I love it even more!

A few years ago, my friend Helen gave me a scoby (a Symbiotic Culture of Bacteria and Yeast), which is used to produce kombucha by fermentation; find out more on page 19. Since then, I have made many, many batches of kombucha and experimented with at least a hundred different flavorings, in what is known as the second fermentation. The great thing about my "kombucha mother" is that it has given me numerous kombucha babies, which I get pleasure in giving to friends as gifts. I send the baby along with lovingly-written instructions on how to look after it so that it can in turn look after my friends and their families.

Long before I got my own scoby, I had seen one when visiting Maria, my grandmother's friend and neighbor, but at the time it did not look very appetizing and I did not like the taste of the tea. Maria drank it on a daily basis, but I remember it being very sour, almost vinegar-like, so perhaps not very appealing to a child. Many years passed before I realized that it is really easy, cheap, and fun to make your own, flavored in any way you like. When I now make my own kombucha, I adapt it to my own taste or to suit my daughter. Thank you, dear Helen, for introducing me to home-made kombucha!

About ten years ago, kombucha started to become more well-known and was sold in bottles for the first time. I drank it happily at fashionable launch parties and glamorous gatherings, along with other delicious, non-alcoholic, healthy drinks. But none of them had anything like the great taste of my own home-made kombucha.

I have made lots of kombucha and learned a lot along the way, but I learned so much more from a really good book that I bought online last year. For anyone who wants to really develop their kombucha skills, I would strongly recommend *The Big Book of Kombucha* by Hannah Crum and Alex LaGory. The authors are real experts and are the people behind KombuchaKamp.com, a site where you can buy scobys and everything else needed to brew kombucha, and also get lots of information and practical advice. Hannah and Alex—I hope we might meet one day over a glass of kombucha!

It takes 8 to 14 days to make your own kombucha with a fresh scoby. The warmer the room, the faster the process—the ideal temperature is 73–84 °F / 23–29 °C. And each time you make kombucha, a new scoby develops.

Successful production depends on good hygiene and good ingredients, and the use of non-chlorinated water. There must be no trace of soap or dishwashing liquid on your hands, jars, bottles, or other equipment.

Glass, wood, and food grade plastic are the best materials to use for making and storing kombucha (I am not keen on plastic myself).

Never use ceramic containers for production or storage, as the acidity may cause the leaching of heavy metals from the ceramic glazes into the liquid. For the same reason, all metals, except stainless steel, are banned.

I make kombucha in 4 or 5-quart (3 or 5-liter) glass jars with taps, so that I can draw some off into a glass when I want to without having to touch the jar. Rinse out your container with hot water (no dishwashing liquid) before you use it. Cleanliness is important.

If you want to take your kombucha really seriously, you can measure its pH level. Kombucha that is ready to drink should have a pH range between 2.5 and 3.5.

Some experts recommend leaving the kombucha to mature for at least five days after decanting it into bottles. Store the kombucha in a cool place or in the fridge. It will keep for at least a year, but will become more acidic over time. Some store-bought versions are extremely acidic, almost vinegar-like.

WHAT CAN GO WRONG?

The main causes of failure when brewing kombucha are traces of antibacterial soap or chemical substances or residue from chemical controls in your ingredients. Mold may appear if the kombucha has the wrong sort of bacterial culture or too little acidification (too high a pH). If your scoby develops mold, the only option is to throw it all away—both the kombucha and the scoby—and start again from the beginning. You will also need to sterilize your jar and let it air for a few days.

You need a vigorous scoby and strong kombucha as your starters. Your kombucha starter must have been allowed to ferment for a minimum of 10 days, ideally at least 14 days. If you use store-bought kombucha to make your first scoby, it must be unpasteurized and unfiltered, ideally plain.

BROWN OR SEE-THROUGH BOTTLES?

Most bottled kombucha is sold in brown bottles which filter out ultraviolet light, which is harmful to the microorganisms. Brown bottles also protect unpasteurized kombucha, enabling it to last longer. I save old-fashioned brown bottles with patent stoppers, and friends aware of my requirements often give them to me as gifts.

HOW LONG DOES KOMBUCHA KEEP?

By law, store-bought kombucha must be stamped with a "best before" date, but its acidity and protective properties mean that it does not really become unfit to drink. However, its taste will change; because the fermentation process continues, it will become increasingly acidic. Flavored kombucha also changes in taste. Home-made, plain kombucha can be kept up to a year, but the longer it is allowed to stand, the more acidic it will become. Flavored versions are best consumed within a couple of months, but I have never kept these longer than a couple of weeks—I just run out.

STORE-BOUGHT KOMBUCHA

It is important that any ready-made kombucha is unpasteurized. Pasteurization removes all the goodness which means the kombucha is then just like any other soft drink, with no probiotic properties at all.

KOMBUCHA YOGURT

My ever-experimenting, health-mad friend Helen suggested I try making kombucha yogurt, something I hadn't thought of doing before she mentioned it. So I tried it, and it worked absolutely fine.

You get different results and consistency with different types of milk. The taste is a little sharper than regular yogurt. All you need is 1 quart or 1 liter of milk of your choice, either animal or plant milk, and a scoby. Equipment-wise, you will need a sterilized glass jar, a clean cotton cloth, and a rubber band to fasten the cloth with. Allow to stand at room temperature for 24 to 36 hours, or, to speed up the process, place in the oven for six to eight hours at 86 °F / 30 °C.

KOMBUCHA — ONLY FOUR INGREDIENTS

WATER

The water must always be boiled. It is best to use spring water that does not contain chlorine, which may be found in tap water. In Sweden we generally have good water, but in many countries the water is highly chlorinated and bactericidal. Also, kombucha is a probiotic drink that should have as much bacterial activity in it as possible. At best, chlorine interferes with the fermentation process of the kombucha, and in the worst case, it kills the scoby.

TEA

You can use various kinds of tea to make kombucha, black, green or white, but beware of teas like Earl Grey that contain essential oils and aromatics. The tea should be organic (chemicals can harm the bacteria culture and, if the worst comes to the worst, you will not get any kombucha) and the content should be 100 percent tealeaves. Always read the label before buying the tea.

Tea for kombucha should draw for a long time, 10–15 minutes with the lid on, so that it secretes enough nitrogen, which the yeast and bacteria culture need in order to grow. Some kombucha experts go so far as to boil the tea for 3–5 minutes, presumably for this very reason. I have tried both and both work.

If you like experimenting it can be fun to try out herbal teas and other kinds of tea, but at your own risk. If there is not enough nitrogen in it you will not get kombucha. Also, there must not be any essential oils in herbal teas and other kinds of tea—the scoby does not like them and in some cases they might kill it off.

When you use herbal teas you are recommended to use 25 percent organic black or green tea to feed the bacteria culture, or alternatively, to use black, white or green tea every third or fourth time you brew kombucha to revitalize your "scoby mother." If you like experimenting, I suggest you have several vigorous scobys in a *Scoby Hotel*, read more on page 20.

I use my lovely Japanese *Satake*-brand cast iron teapots, which are very good for tea that has to draw for a long time, because they retain the heat and make it easier for all the useful substances to come out of the tealeaves. I prefer the taste of classic black tea in my kombucha, but you should try things out until you find your favorite flavor.

SUGAR

Brewing kombucha needs a source of sugar. This is to feed the microorganisms in the kombucha culture, not us, and the final sugar content of the drink is low. You could say that the sugar is eaten up by the yeast and converted into the constituents of the drink. Tea blends with low sugar content (fewer carbohydrates) will release fewer active substances—if you cut down on the amount of sugar your scoby will starve, the kombucha will be weak and mold may form.

I use organic brown GMO-free cane sugar, but any cane sugar will do. Some experts maintain that organic white sugar is better, because that type of sugar is easier for the microorganisms to assimilate.

You can also use other sources of sugar, for example honey (please avoid RAW honey, which contains natural antibacterial substances that may inhibit the growth of the kombucha culture), molasses, coconut palm sugar, agave syrup, maple syrup, brown rice syrup, glucose, dextrose, etc., but then you cannot be sure of getting the same even quality in the finished product. This is because the composition of these types of sugar varies and it is harder for the kombucha culture to access the nutriment. In addition unpleasant pungent, bitter, or sour after-tastes may be produced.

Stevia, Xylitol, fructose-glucose syrup and all other artificial sweeteners are not suitable for brewing kombucha.

SCOBY

See page 19.

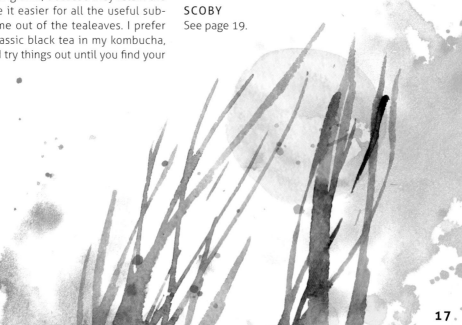

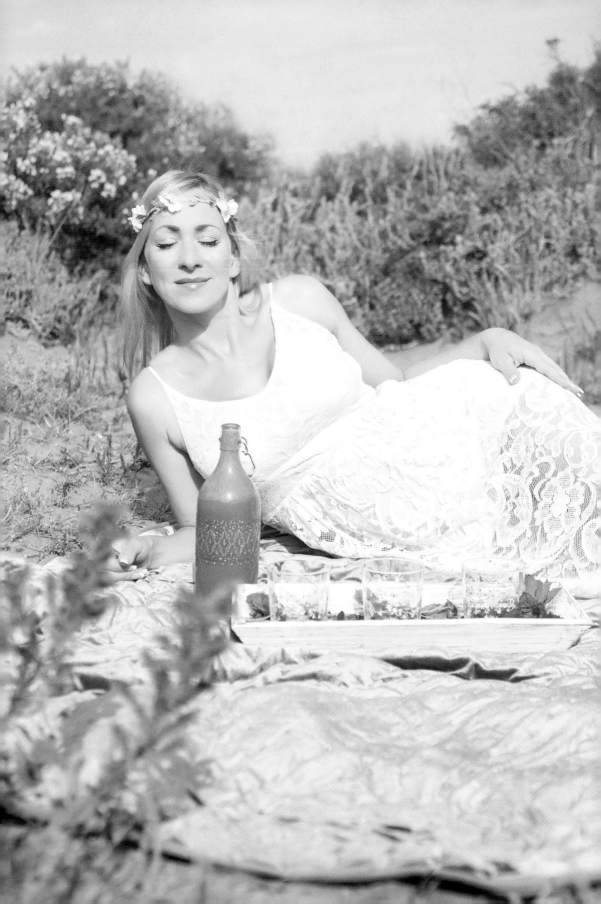

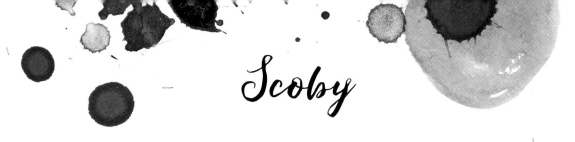

Scoby

Scoby stands for Symbiothic Colony Of Bacteria and Yeast. SCOBY is often called a fungus, but in fact it is not a fungus but a symbiosis of yeast fungi and lactic acid bacteria. It has many names—scoby, kombucha culture, kombucha fungus, volga fingus, tea fungus and Kombucha Mother—and it is used for making Kombucha tea. The scoby can vary in color from pale and transparent to more like tea-brown, depending on which tea you use and how old the scoby is. The older it is, the darker and less potent it becomes. A new scoby is white, slightly yellowish or almost transparent. An older scoby has something brown and muddy-looking around it, and this is yeast.

MAKE YOUR OWN SCOBY

You can start your very own scoby (kombucha culture) from scratch in a few weeks with just a few ingredients by following the instructions on page 21. Remember that hygiene is important and the choice of ingredients will determine how successful you are, and that the water must not contain chlorine. There must be no traces of soap or dishwashing liquid left either on your hands or on the equipment, jars, or bottles. Towels and cotton cloths to be used for covering the jar must be clean. The cloth must be thick enough to keep out flies, dust, other bacterial cultures, and any other undesirables, but not too thick, because air must still be able to get in. It is a good idea to rub or wash your hands with a tablespoon of finished kombucha after washing them if you are going to handle a SCOBY, so as not to disturb it. It is best to make kombucha in glass jars.

FRESH, FROZEN, OR DRIED?

If you cannot or do not want to make your own, you can order it online, but check first with your friends or on Facebook whether any of them are experienced kombucha brewers and can share with you. There are also various Facebook groups who share their kombucha babies for free.

If you buy one, you are always recommended to go for a fresh scoby that has not been kept in a fridge, freeze-dried, dried or frozen, because anything other than a fresh scoby produces a much weaker fermentation, and that increases the risk of mold. The size of the scoby is also important, so check that it is full size and not a miniature made in a small test tube to reduce production costs, because again this will result in inadequate fermentation and a risk of mold. When you start the kombucha, you need an environment that is acidic enough for the good bacteria to be able to grow well and no unwanted mold will form.

Fresh scoby is usually sent in a padded envelope, together with the instructions and a little kombucha tea, which is to be used together with the scoby to provide an acidic environment for good fermentation. The scoby must be dealt with immediately on arrival, but first just let it get to room temperature in its packaging if it has been cold. When it is delivered you need to have organic sugar and organic tea at home, as the bacteria culture will be harmed by traces of biocides. Make sure it is not left outside when it is too hot or too cold, in direct sun or below freezing!

SENSITIVE TO HEAT AND COLD

The scoby is sensitive to both heat and cold and thrives best at just above room temperature, between 73 and 84 °F or 23 and 29 °C. The lower the room temperature, the slower the fermentation. The warmer the kombucha culture, the faster the process will go, but temperatures of 85 °F (30 °C) and above are not recommended.

Strong, direct sunlight is harmful to kombucha, as for all other fermentation. The scoby must never be placed in hot tea above 108 °F (42 °C), as this will weaken it or, in the worst case, kill it. Never keep the scoby in the fridge, because this will weaken it and risk killing it. Even if it survives the cold it will not produce a proper fermentation and this usually leads to mold. The scoby can cope with the cold for a short time, for example during transport, but it will need time to recover at room temperature in its liquid.

TO RINSE OR NOT TO RINSE?

A scoby should not normally be rinsed in water, because the bacterial culture will be weakened and may become unbalanced, which means your next kombucha could be moldy. However, if you choose to do so for some reason, for instance if there is a lot of yeast around the scoby, you should immediately put it in strong, ready-made kombucha for twenty-four hours or more so that it can recover before new brewing.

FLOAT OR SINK?

When you put the ready-made scoby into the sweet tea to ferment your kombucha tea, it may float at the top, hover in the middle or, most commonly, sink to the bottom—all of these are normal. Wherever the *Kombucha Mother* is in the jar, it will grow a new baby scoby on the surface. The *Mother Scoby* may or may not grow along with the baby—both are normal. And it is easy to separate them if you want to give one away or start several kombuchas at the same time.

SCOBY HOTEL

If you are going to keep your leftover or extra scobys, new or old, for presents, or you just do not want to be continually brewing kombucha at home, the scoby should be kept in a glass jar with ready-made kombucha in it, a so-called *Kombucha Hotel*, never in the fridge, because the cold will weaken the scoby and there will be a risk of mold in future kombucha brewing. For your scobys to thrive, their environment must have a pH of 2.5–3.5. You can keep them for up to six months in their protective environment at room temperature, away from direct sunlight, covered with a thick, clean cotton cloth fastened with a rubber band. Have a quick look at them from time to time and mix in a little sweet tea every month or every other month when the level of the liquid gets low. If a lot of yeast builds up, you can filter it off, because the yeast may harm the scoby culture.

WHAT CAN YOU DO WITH LEFTOVER SCOBY?

There are lots of tips on the internet for leftover scoby—there are even companies that make skin care products from scoby, from rejuvenating face masks, creams, plasters for all kinds of wounds, doggy treats, fruit jellies, sushi, or meat substitutes, and everything in between. Leftover scoby can simply be added to compost. Or you could share your scoby babies with your friends!

GIVE THEM AWAY AS PRESENTS

Your scoby will grow quickly if it is happy living with you. With every new kombucha, you get a new scoby as well. In perfect conditions a new scoby can be produced after ten days —a thin skin forms on the tea's surface, like a transparent jelly that gets thicker and stronger every day.

To give a scoby away as a present, pick it up with a spoon or tongs made of stainless steel, plastic, or wood—or clean hands (preferably washed with 1 tablespoon of ready-made kombucha), place it in a wide-mouthed glass jar with enough ready-made kombucha to cover it and put on the lid. You can use double reclosable, thick, BPA-free plastic bags if the scoby is to be kept for a short time, but it is important that the liquid should cover it and accompany it as part of the present.

The scoby can grow enormous and last for several years if you want to use the same one, but I swap a small one for a fresh one every now and then. If you want to give away a substantial scoby, you can also cut it to the right size if it has grown too big or divide it up in different ways. I always give away fresh, new scoby babies, because they look more appetizing—well, a scoby looks pretty unappetizing, especially an old one.

DRINK A TOAST IN FLAVORED, BUBBLING KOMBUCHA — SECOND FERMENTATION

I like plain kombucha without flavoring, and it is really nice in smoothies—but lemonade-like flavored drinks made from kombucha with fruits, berries, spices, and herbs have a special place in my heart. Also you can use them in smoothies instead of plain kombucha; the ones made with spices and herbs work particularly well.

The second fermentation is great fun, easy, and incredibly good. It is so cool, I come over all lyrical just at the thought of trying out new flavors.

You can flavor the kombucha with fruit, berries, herbs, leaves, roots, or edible flowers—but always be scrupulous about cleaning them. The fruit and berries can be chopped, pureed, freeze-dried, dried, pulverized, frozen, or as juice. Let it draw for a few days at room temperature until it gets a little bit of carbonic acid and a wonderful taste, then put the bottles in the fridge. If you are going to keep flavored kombucha in the fridge for longer than a few days it is best to strain it, as then the fermentation will stop.

Use no more than 1 tablespoon of fruit to 2 cups (500 ml) of kombucha. Herbs and spices do not contain sugar and can be used a bit more generously. Try it out until you get the taste you want.

Safety Tips

When brewing kombucha with flavoring, you always do it in two stages of fermentation:

♥ The first happens while it is developing in the glass jar with scoby.

♥ The second happens when it is ready and you pour it off into tightly-corked bottles or jars and leave it to stand at room temperature for a few days, before putting it in the fridge. The warmer it is, the faster the process goes. You flavor the kombucha during the second phase.

If you want to avoid cleaning up—or in the worst case repainting—the entire kitchen and everything within reach, there are a few rules to be followed if you do the second fermentation/ flavoring in bottles.

♥ The glass bottles must be sterilized with boiling water, there must be no traces of dishwasher liquid left.

♥ The glass bottles <u>must</u> be pressure-resistant and have a tight-fitting cork (not metal), otherwise there is a risk of the bottles exploding. For safety's sake you can keep the bottles in a closed box, for instance a picnic coolbox so there will be minimal damage and cleaning up if the bottles do explode.

♥ You need to release the pressure now and then. It is a good idea to wrap a clean towel round the top of the bottle while opening it very carefully a little at a time.

♥ Only use a little of the flavoring (5–10%) to be fermented, mainly because too much sweet fruit produces a lot of gas, so when you open it all the contents will spray out before you have had a chance to taste it. I promise, I have tried it. The more fruit, the greater the risk of hours of cleaning up. I have had to scrub the kitchen from floor to ceiling countless times, and repainted it on a number of occasions. Blueberry kombucha is not to be trifled with! Be extra careful with purees and dried fruits that have a lot of sugar in them. I usually have no more than 1 tablespoon of fruit, berries, or puree per 2-cup (500 ml) bottle. With spices, herbs, and lemon peel you can use more, because they do not contain sugar.

♥ Never shake the bottle or run around with it before it is to be opened. It is a carbonated drink and, just like champagne or any other sparkling drink, you have to handle it carefully.

♥ Keeping the kombucha in the fridge for a few hours before opening makes it easier.

♥ For a party or some other kind of celebration, open the bottles yourself and stand them on the table, or pour the kombucha into jugs, otherwise the guests may get a bottle sprayed over them. (Kyle, I am sorry your shirt was ruined just before your speech at Osteo-Strong's opening banquet. Lucky you had an extra shirt with you!)

♥ If you want safer preparation, less washing up and to keep flavored kombucha for a bit longer, you can flavor it directly in the big jar you did the first fermentation in. Do not forget to remove the scoby and starter liquid for the next kombucha, and screw the lid on if you want bubbles. The wider the opening, the smaller the risk of spraying contents. If you do it that way, you can use a little more flavoring, strain the kombucha after 2–4 days and keep it in pressure-resistant bottles.

Suggested flavorings

Below are some of my favorites, calculated for 2 cups or 500 ml of kombucha.

- ♥ 1 tbsp berries of your choice or crushed/diced fruit, juice, or puree

- ♥ 1–2 tbsp mixed spices, herbs, or herbal tea

- ♥ **Vanilla** (1 pinch vanilla powder or ½ vanilla bean, cut in half and with the seeds scraped out)

- ♥ **Minty Raspberry** (1 tbsp crushed raspberries, 1 tbsp chopped mint)

- ♥ **Ginger Fire** (¾ –1 in or 2–3 cm organic ginger, thinly sliced)

- ♥ **Wild Vanilla Blueberry** (1 tbsp wild, fresh or frozen and defrosted blueberries, 1 pinch vanilla powder)

- ♥ **Apple Pie** (1 tbsp apple juice and ½ tsp cinnamon or chai spice mix)

- ♥ **Turmeric Touch** (1–2 pieces fresh, organic turmeric, thinly sliced)

- ♥ **Strawberry Banana** (2 tbsp mashed banana, 1 tbsp diced or crushed strawberries)

- ♥ **Choco Banana** (2 tbsp mashed banana, 1 tsp raw cocoa powder)

- ♥ **Apricot Rose** (1 fresh, sliced apricot, 1 tbsp rose petals)

- ♥ **Master Cleanse** (¼ diced apple, 1 pinch grated lime zest, 2 tbsp real maple syrup, one pinch chili powder)

- ♥ **Cranberry Vanilla** (1 tbsp fresh or frozen cranberries or lingonberries, 1 pinch vanilla powder) **Hot Date** (1 large or 2 small dates, chopped, 1 pinch cayenne pepper)

- ♥ **Black Beauty** (4–5 blackberries crushed or in pieces, 1 pinch vanilla powder)

- ♥ **Turkish Coffee** (1 date, chopped, 1 tbsp strong coffee or 1 tsp organic coffee powder, one pinch ground cardamom)

- ♥ **Cold Fighter** (1 tsp sea buckthorn powder, ½–1 in / 1–2 cm fresh ginger and 1 piece fresh turmeric, thinly sliced)

- ♥ **Christmas Kombucha** (1 tsp gingerbread spice mix or 1 tsp mixed whole dried spices: black pepper, cloves, cinnamon stick, bitter orange peel)

- ♥ **Papaya Passion** (1 tbsp papaya nectar or crushed papaya, 1 pinch lemon zest, 1 tsp passion fruit juice)

- ♥ **Pina Colada** (1 tbsp chopped pineapple, 1 tsp shredded coconut)

- ♥ **Tropical Delight** (1 tbsp pineapple juice, 1 tbsp chopped mango, 1 tsp fresh passion fruit juice)

- ♥ **Passionberry** (2 tbsp fresh passion fruit juice, 1 tsp crushed raspberries, 1 pinch lime zest)

- ♥ **Raisin Cookie** (1 tbsp organic raisins, 1 pinch ground cinnamon, 1 pinch vanilla powder)

- ♥ **Rhubarb Pie** (1 tbsp rhubarb, chopped, 1 pinch cinnamon, 1 pinch cardamom)

- ♥ **Rosehipnotic** (1 tbsp dried rose hips, 1 tbsp rose petals)

- ♥ **Superbuzz** (1 tsp honey, 1 tsp bee pollen, 1 tsp maca powder, 1 tsp chamomile, dried flowers)

- ♥ **Goji Delight** (1 tbsp dried goji berries, ½ in / 1 cm ginger, thinly sliced)

- ♥ **Mochabucha** (1 pinch raw cocoa powder, 1 tsp organic coffee powder)

- ♥ **Pepperbeet** (1 pinch ground black pepper, 1 tbsp fresh beetroot, diced)

- ♥ **Spicy Carrot** (1 tbsp freshly-squeezed carrot juice, 1 pinch cayenne pepper)

- ♥ **Virgin Mojito** (1 tbsp mint, ½ tsp lime zest)

- ♥ **Orange Blastoff** (1 tbsp freshly-squeezed orange juice, 1 pinch ground cinnamon, 1 piece fresh turmeric, thinly sliced)

- ♥ **Citrus Kick** (1 tbsp freshly-squeezed mandarin or orange juice, ½ tsp mandarin or orange zest, a few orage flowers)

- ♥ **Sweet Licorice** (1 tbsp dried, ground licorice root, 1 tsp honey)

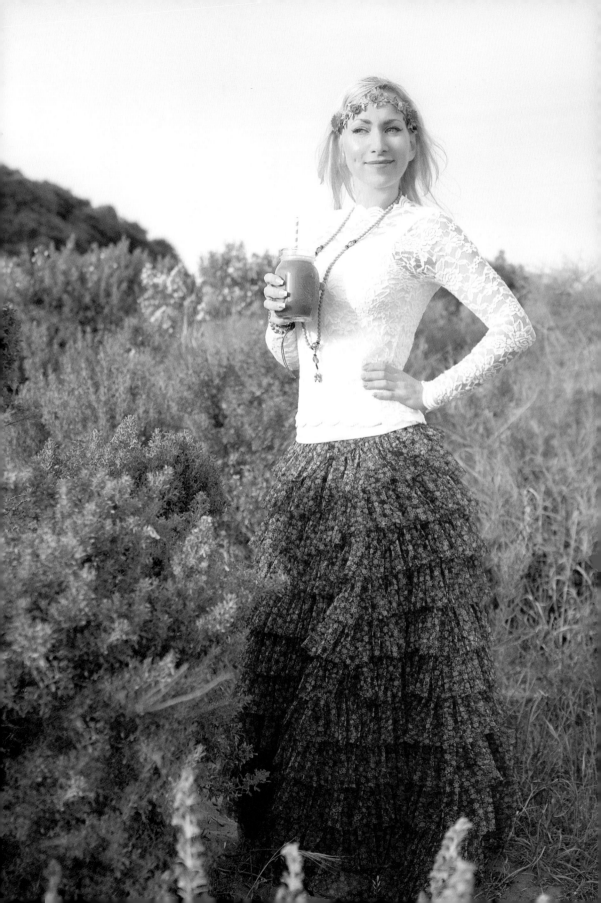

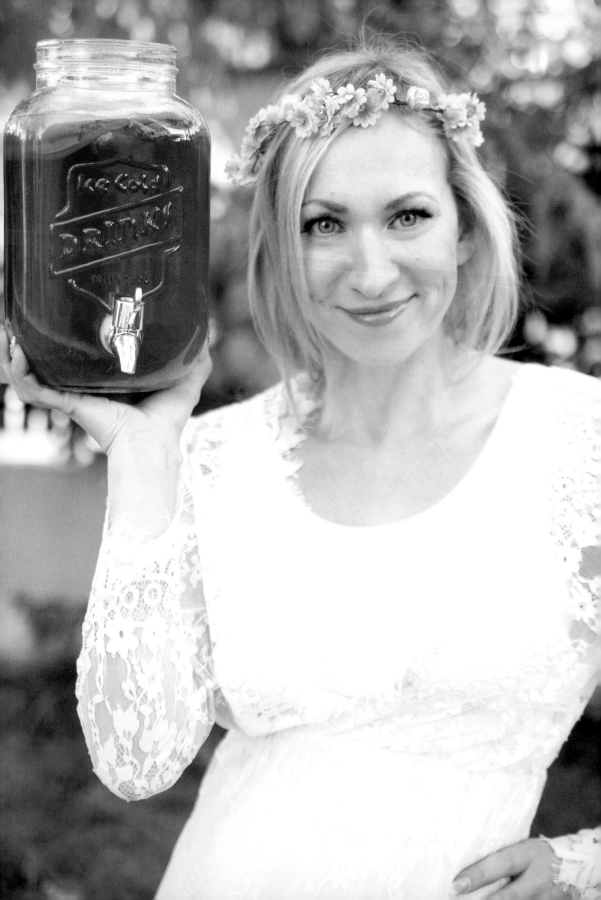

Scoby – METHOD

YOU WILL NEED:

- ♥ 1 tbsp / 3–4 teabags organic black tea (green and white tea will do too)
- ♥ 1 quart / 1 liter water, preferably spring water
- ♥ 3½ tbsp / 50 ml or 1¾ oz / 45–50 g organic cane sugar
- ♥ a bottle of unpasteurized, unfiltered ready-made kombucha
- ♥ teapot, cast iron would be good
- ♥ kitchen equipment (saucepan, strainer, spoon, ladle, knife, funnel)
- ♥ a glass container with a wide mouth, at least 1½ quarts or 1.5 liters
- ♥ thick cotton cloth or kitchen towel and rubber band
- ♥ pressure-resistant bottles with tight-fitting corks

METHOD:

1. **CLEAN THE EQUIPMENT.** Start by washing all your equipment carefully, making sure you rinse off any traces of dishwashing liquid. As with all fermentation it is important to think about hygiene, otherwise bad bacteria may increase. I usually disinfect my glass jars with boiling water, because no chemicals or traces of chemicals should remain.

2. **USE STRONG TEA.** Boil the water and pour it over the tealeaves/teabags in the pot. Tea for kombucha should be allowed to draw for a long time, 10–15 minutes with the lid on so that it secretes enough nitrogen, which the yeast and bacteria culture need in order to grow. Some experts and Kombucha manufacturers recommend boiling the tea for a few minutes to get extra strong mineral content and nitrogen in the tea. Strain out the tealeaves if you used loose tea, or remove the teabags if you used those, and add the sugar, which must be dissolved completely. The sugar will feed the culture, so very little will be left in the finished drink.

3. **COOL DOWN.** Let the tea cool down to room temperature or a maximum of 104 °F or 40 °C. To speed up the cooling process you can put the covered saucepan in cold water.

4. **ADD THE KOMBUCHA.** Pour the tea into glass jars or containers and then add a whole bottle of unpasteurized kombucha to the tea. The proportion of tea to kombucha should be between 3:1 and 5:1, i.e., three to five times as much tea as kombucha. Cover the container with cotton cloth or a clean kitchen towel, and fasten it in place with a rubber band to protect it from flies, dust, and other undesirables.

5. **FERMENT.** Place the container in a warm, sheltered spot. The ideal temperature is a few degrees above room temperature, 73–84 °F or 23–29 °C. Strong and direct sunlight is harmful to the kombucha, like all other fermentations. Leave to stand for 3 to 4 weeks, until a ¼– ½ in / ½ –1 cm thick layer of SCOBY/kombucha culture has formed on the surface and the tea has acquired a slightly vinegary aroma (do not touch it during this time). The scoby is now ready to be used for your home-made kombucha in large quantities.

6. **REMOVE THE SCOBY** (the kombucha fungus) with clean utensils or clean hands. Leave no traces of soap on your hands, and it is a good idea to wash your hands with 1 tablespoon of ready-made kombucha before you touch it. Place it temporarily in a small glass jar while you clean your large container to start a new kombucha.

7. **POUR INTO BOTTLES.** Reserve ¾ cup or 200 ml for a new kombucha (Nb: Not from the bottom.). I usually use about 10% of ready-made kombucha to lukewarm sweet tea and put the scoby in it. Pour the remainder of the kombucha into the bottle, through a strainer if you want to get rid of most of the muddiness. Now you can do a so-called *second fermentation* and flavor the kombucha or leave it plain.

8. **STORE.** Store the drink in a cool place or in the fridge, preferably in the dark or in a dark glass bottle. It will keep for at least a year in these conditions (it will get more acidic as time goes on) but my kombucha gets used up within a week! Read more about Kombucha on page 15.

9. **MAKE A NEW KOMBUCHA.** Use the scoby and the liquid you reserved to brew new kombucha. That means going through the process again from step 1, but instead of adding a bottle of bought kombucha in step 4, use your own home-brewed Kombucha plus the scoby you grew, see page 26. When the scoby has grown a little, you will need to use a few drops of ready-made kombucha plus scoby to start the process.

Plain Kombucha

YOU WILL NEED:

- ♥ 2 tbsp / 6–8 teabags organic black tea (green and white tea will do too)
- ♥ 2 quarts / 2 liters water, preferably spring water
- ♥ 7 tbsp / 100 ml or 3–3 ½ oz or 90–100 g organic cane sugar
- ♥ one kombucha culture (SCOBY)
- ♥ ¾ cup / 200 ml ready-made, unfiltered, unpasteurized kombucha
- ♥ teapot, cast iron would be good
- ♥ kitchen equipment (saucepan, strainer, spoon, ladle, knife, funnel)
- ♥ a glass container with a wide mouth, at least 2 ½ quarts or 2.5 liters
- ♥ thick cotton cloth or kitchen towel and rubber band
- ♥ pressure-resistant bottles with tight-fitting corks

METHOD:

1. **CLEAN THE EQUIPMENT.** Start by washing all your equipment carefully, making sure you rinse off any traces of dishwashing liquid. As with all fermentation it is important to think about hygiene, otherwise bad bacteria may increase. I usually disinfect my glass jars with boiling water.

2. **USE STRONG TEA.** Boil the water and pour it over the tealeaves/teabags in the pot. Tea for kombucha should be allowed to draw for a long time, 10–15 minutes with the lid on so that it secretes enough nitrogen, which the yeast and bacteria culture need in order to grow. Some experts and Kombucha manufacturers recommend boiling the tea for a few minutes to get extra strong mineral content and nitrogen in the tea. Strain out the tealeaves if you used loose tea, or remove the teabags if you used those, and add the sugar, which must be dissolved completely. The sugar will feed the culture, so very little will be left in the finished drink.

3. **COOL DOWN.** Let the tea cool down to room temperature or a maximum of 108 °F or 42 °C. To speed up the cooling process you can put the covered saucepan in cold water.

4. **ADD THE KOMBUCHA.** Pour the tea into the container and then add the ready-made kombucha to the tea, stir, and add the SCOBY (the kombucha culture). (If you are making kombucha tea for the first time, you should add the

scoby together with the liquid you got with it.) The proportion of tea to kombucha should be at least 10:1, i.e. at least ten times as much tea as kombucha. This is important in order to get the fermentation process off to a good start. In this way, the tea also protects it from harmful micro-organisms, as no harmful bacteria can develop in the acidic environment. Cover the container with cotton cloth or a clean kitchen towel fasten it in place with a rubber band to protect it from flies, dust, and other undesirables.

5. **FERMENT.** Place the container in a warm, sheltered spot. The ideal temperature is a few degrees above room temperature. Strong and direct sunlight is harmful to the kombucha, like all other fermentations. Leave for at least 8–14 days, and the warmer it is the faster the process will go. The ideal temperature is 73–84 °F / 23–29 °C.

6. **REMOVE THE SCOBY** (the kombucha fungus) with tongs or clean hands. (Nb: No traces of soap), and place it temporarily in a small glass jar while you clean your large container to start a new kombucha. If necessary, you can rinse it carefully under cold or lukewarm running water, but then it must stand for at least twenty-four hours in ready-made kombucha in order to recover.

7. **POUR INTO BOTTLES.** Reserve ¾ cup or 200 ml for a new kombucha. I usually use about 10 % of ready-made kombucha to lukewarm sweet tea and put the scoby in it. Pour the remainder of the kombucha into the bottle, then you can do a so-called *second fermentation* and flavor the kombucha or leave it plain. Clean the flavoring and cut it in small pieces. Add the flavoring to the bottle, close it, and leave to stand for 3 to 5 days in a warm dark place. Then keep the bottles in the fridge. Enjoy!

8. **STORE.** Store the drink cool in the fridge, preferably in the dark or in dark glass bottles. It will keep for at least a year in these conditions, but my kombucha gets used up within a week! Read more about Kombucha on page 15.

9. **MAKE A NEW KOMBUCHA.** Use the scoby and the liquid you reserved to brew new kombucha. That means going through the process again from step 1, but instead of adding a bottle of bought kombucha in step 4, use your own home-brewed Kombucha plus the scoby you grew. When the scoby has grown a little, you will need to use a few drops of ready-made kombucha plus scoby to start the process.

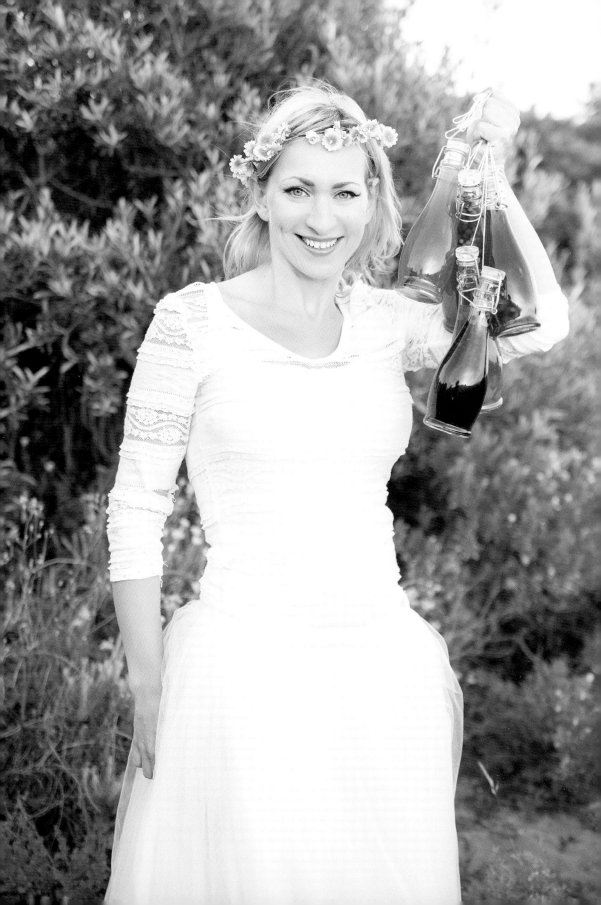

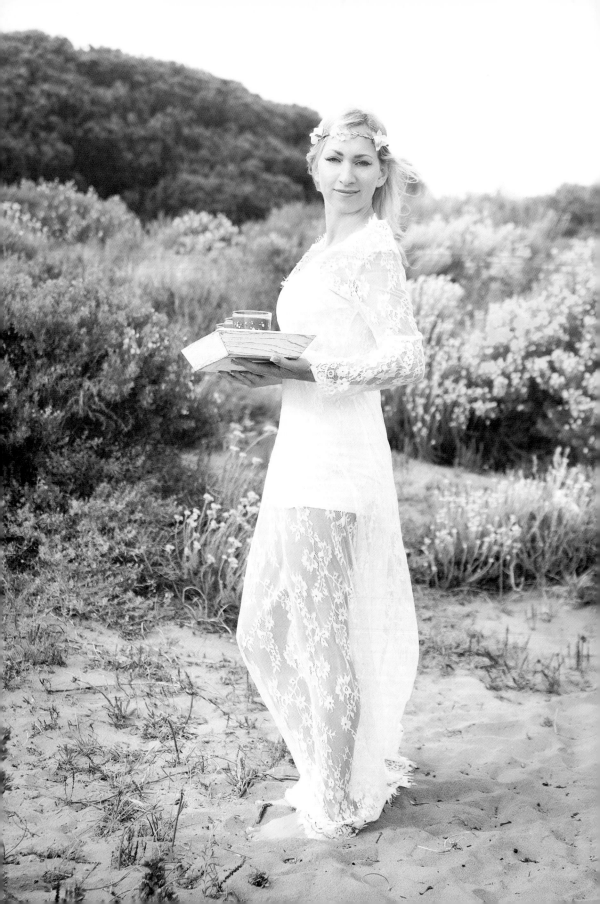

Kefir

For me, kefir means a nostalgia trip back to my childhood in Soviet Estonia in the 1980s and early 1990s. My beloved grandmother was in the habit of making her own soured or cultured milk. We had no access to yogurt culture, and it was a matter of luck if kefir was available in the stores, as the shelves were mostly empty. But old Maria, my grandmother's neighbor and friend, made her own kefir.

When I was 4 or 5, I would mash strawberries, blueberries, blackcurrants, raspberries, and other treats from my grandmother's garden into my kefir, or my soured or cultured milk. There was sometimes honey from a neighbor's hive. I have realized now that these were my first smoothies—not so smooth, made with just a fork, but still smoothies.

Maria has a special place in my heart. She had a lengthy, adventurous, exciting, tragic, and sad tale to tell about how she and all her family, including a new baby daughter and two small boys, were deported to Siberia in the 1940s in the middle of a cold night in early spring, and how they lived there for many years. Her story has had a permanent influence on the way I view life. Maria taught me how to survive on virtually nothing. And she was very definitely a survivor herself, living until the age of 93. She did not stop riding her bike until she was 90.

I am grateful to her for teaching me to bake and appreciate black rye bread, made with real sourdough, and for showing me how to make kefir. She gave me tea made from tea fungus (kombucha), which I did not appreciate very much at the time. And she gave me kvass to try as well as many other delicious, healthy things she always had in her house. I wish now that I could ask her all the questions that have arisen since she died—it is not until now, long after her death, that I realize how much she wanted to teach me.

Another thing I have Maria to thank for is something that I now absolutely love and am almost addicted to (my friends will vouch for the fact that I eat it at least three times a week)—buckwheat. Maria used to go around chewing on raw buckwheat grain that she kept in her pocket. When I asked her why, she said that that was how she and her family had survived all those years in the cold of Siberia, where nothing grew and the temperatures in winter could fall to below minus 40 degrees. Thank you, lovely Maria, wherever you are, for all the knowledge I carry with me. I hope it will now be useful to other people.

HEALTH-PROMOTING PROPERTIES

Kefir is a fermented milk drink with a slightly sour taste that can be lightly carbonated. It has its origins in the Caucasus mountains and is said to be the secret behind the excellent health enjoyed by the local population in their old age. Kefir has been a popular drink in Russia and other Eastern European countries for the last hundred years, and these days it is known across half the world. Kefir grains are shrouded in myth, and, although there are a number of traditional stories involving the supernatural, there is no actual historical evidence of their origins.

Unfortunately, store-bought kefir is often pasteurized, has very little variety in its bacterial strains, and also has a lot of added sugar, which means it is not as healthy as it could be. But, luckily, making your own kefir is very easy.

Kefir can be useful for those people who suffer from ulcerative colitis or IBS, as kefir has been shown to downregulate inflammation in the gut and increase production of anti-inflammatory cytokines (proteins) that can keep the inflammation in check. And because the skin mirrors the digestive tract, kefir can also help combat eczema, acne, and rosacea, and soothe the effects of allergic reactions.

Kefir has a naturally low lactose content and has also been shown to facilitate the breakdown of lactose in people who are lactose intolerant.

In addition, kefir has antibacterial properties and so can help combat fungal infections. Vaginal candida infection is a health problem for many women, caused partly by lifestyle and acidification of the body. My grandmother recommended that I apply kefir direct to the vagina. Much later, some midwives gave me the tip of dipping my tampons into kefir or yogurt, but most tampons are bleached with chemicals and so this cannot necessarily be recommended.

While I was growing up, kefir or soured cream were used to treat minor burns such as sunburn. Our grandmothers and their grandmothers knew a great many things that have now been lost to us. Imagine if we could go back in time and benefit from the wisdom of all those amazing women.

MICROORGANISMS

Home-made kefir contains a range of different types of microorganism in the form of yeasts and beneficial bacteria. It contains over fifty types of good strains of bacteria, while "regular" store-bought yogurt only has seven. What is more, the latter only live in the body for one day, whereas the good bacteria in home-made kefir can survive for much longer, and can even survive treatment with antibiotics. The yeast has an important role to play in digestion and in keeping out intruders.

In addition to useful bacteria and yeast, kefir contains vitamins, minerals, proteins, amino acids, enzymes, prebiotics, and probiotics. It is rich in thiamine, vitamin B12, folate, vitamin K2, and also calcium, magnesium, and phosphorus.

Along with kombucha, it is probably one of the most potent probiotic foods in existence. Find out more about kombucha on page 15.

THINGS YOU WILL NEED TO BUY

KEFIR GRAINS

Milk and water kefir grains can be bought online, where you can also source the equipment and other items needed. If you are lucky, you will be able to obtain a starter culture from someone who already has fermented kefir grains (since the grains grow continuously). There are groups on Facebook that sell grains or share them free of charge. The same applies to kombucha/scoby.

With dried kefir grains, it takes longer to make the kefir as you have to activate the grains first.

EQUIPMENT

Your utensils must be stainless steel; any other metal can leach out into the kefir and could, in the worst-case scenario, poison the grains. Clean glass jars and clean towels are essential. The whey should be strained through a cheesecloth, a coffee filter, or, better still, a nylon strainer, which will not damage the grain. If the grains are large, they can be removed from the whey using a wooden ladle or stainless-steel spoon.

ACTIVATING DRIED KEFIR GRAINS

Kefir is made from milk or water and kefir grains. The starter culture looks like a clump of grain and consists of bacteria, yeast, salt, protein, lipids, and sugar, which the bacteria feed on.

MILK KEFIR GRAINS

Dried milk kefir grains are activated in fresh milk. The first batch will take three to seven days, then kefir will be produced every 18 to 48 hours. Fermentation takes place at room temperature, and the grain can be reused for many years.

Start the fermentation process by adding 3 to 4 tablespoons of grains to a jar holding about 1¼ cups / 300 ml of pasteurized milk. Cover with a thin cotton cloth and fasten with a rubber band. Change the milk every day as the grains need plenty of lactose to feed on. The milk you strain off is suitable for consumption provided it does not smell or taste unpleasant. Keep changing the milk until the milk in the jar starts to thicken, smell sour, and separate from the whey. If the temperature in the room is low, it may take 2 to 4 weeks before the grains start producing kefir, so be patient.

Be aware that over the first few days the milk might smell of yeast and froth a little at the surface, but within three to seven days the microorganisms should have stabilized. The kefir should then smell sour and slightly yeasty.

WATER KEFIR GRAINS

Dried water kefir grains are activated in fresh water, a process that normally takes 3 to 4 days. After that, the grains will produce kefir every 24 to 48 hours. Two teaspoons of dried grains make 3 to 4 tablespoons of activated grains, which will ferment up to about 2 quarts / 2 liters of water kefir. Fermentation takes place at room temperature, and the grain can then be reused for many years.

Start by dissolving 4 tablespoons of sugar in a generous ¾ cup / 200 ml of hot water. Add cold water until you have 1 quart or 1 liter of

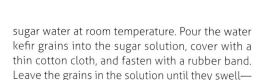

sugar water at room temperature. Pour the water kefir grains into the sugar solution, cover with a thin cotton cloth, and fasten with a rubber band. Leave the grains in the solution until they swell—no more than four days.

If nothing happens after four days, start again with the same grains and some fresh sugar water.

SHOULD I RINSE MY GRAINS?

Activated kefir grains do not need to be rinsed, they are happiest sitting in their milk. But if they have acquired fat deposits or have gone too long without a top-up so that they are beginning to run out of food or develop the wrong type of sourness, you may want to rinse them, and preferably in milk. You can also rinse in water at room temperature, but the water must not be too warm as this will kill them.

KEFIR GRAINS CANNOT WITHSTAND COLD OR HEAT

Kefir is happiest at normal room temperature, up to 100 °F / 40 °C. The higher the temperature, the faster the process. Never heat your kefir grains, and make sure any thermos you use is not too hot. When the grains are not "working," keep them at the top of the fridge where it is warmest. Remember that the grains will suffer if the temperature in the fridge is below 46 °F / 8 °C and will start to die.

THE GRAINS ARE MULTIPLYING—WHAT DO I DO?

Just make more kefir, give some away to friends, or sell some on the internet. Or try eating the grains—they are better probiotics than the kefir itself.

GOING AWAY? TAKING A BREAK?

If it is just for a weekend or up to a week, the grains will keep in a container in the fridge. Fill the container with milk or store-bought kefir and place it at the top of the fridge where it is warmest. You will not need very much milk for a weekend, but if you are away for a week, add the same quantity as you would normally—see page 35.

If you are away for a longer period, you have two options.

FREEZING: Rinse and allow the grains to dry for a while, preferably patting them dry with paper towels or a clean kitchen towel. Put them in the freezer together with some powdered milk. The

powdered milk will protect the grains against freezer burn. The grains will keep this way for two or three months, often longer. Revive them by defrosting them and rinsing in water at room temperature, and then start a batch of kefir as normal.

DRYING: Rinse and allow the grains to dry completely; this will take one or two days. Place the grains in a bag with some dried milk, so that they can "float" in the powder. They are said to keep for one to two years this way. Revive the grains by placing them in milk, changing it every day until they have regained their proper size. Start a batch of kefir as normal. It might take a few batches before the grains are working at their optimum capacity. You can also allow the grains to grow back to their normal size in water at room temperature, and then start with milk again.

MILK KEFIR

Kefir made from milk is the most common type, and generally speaking it can be made from any kind of milk: animal milk from cows, goats, sheep, or camels, preferably unpasteurized, or plant milk such as coconut milk. Milk kefir grains ferment the milk to produce a kefir drink that is similar to yogurt. If you want your kefir to be creamier, add a dash of cream. The more kefir grains you have, the quicker the result.

UNPASTEURIZED V PASTEURIZED MILK

Choose organic milk for preference. The easiest way is to start with pasteurized whole milk, but do not use UHT as it is "dead" milk. Unhomogenized milk is a bit more difficult to work with, and the trickiest is fresh, unpasteurized milk, which is guaranteed to produce the creamiest, most delicious kefir of them all and most resembles the original. The difficult part is probably dealing with the fat in unhomogenized milk and the bacterial flora in unpasteurized versions.

Do not change from one type of milk to another too abruptly, particularly if changing from pasteurized whole milk to a "better" type. Contrary to what you might think, these can seem a bit more problematic to begin with, perhaps because they have not been broken down.

Unpasteurized milk has a lot of lactic acid bacteria of its own that may compete with the bacteria in the kefir. Start by introducing a quarter of unpasteurized milk to three quarters pasteurized. Once that mixture has turned into kefir, you can swap out another quarter of the pasteurized milk. Continue in this way until the process works with just unpasteurized milk. Hold some grains back and keep feeding them with pasteurized milk, in case the grains in the unpasteurized milk are outcompeted by the milk's own bacteria. You should not have a problem reversing the substitution process if necessary.

WATER KEFIR

You can also make kefir from water, e.g. from spring water, purified or filtered fresh water, or even from coconut water. So if you are not a lover of dairy products, you have the option of water kefir instead. NB: The grains for water kefir are not the same as those for milk kefir. Water kefir normally has a lower concentration of the microorganisms that are good for the stomach, so you should drink even more of it.

Water kefir grains ferment fresh water or coconut water into a drink called water kefir. It is a good idea to add a few drops of mineral water to the water, as water kefir likes water with nutrients.

Note that water kefir contains a lot of living microorganisms from the outset, but it can take a couple of months before it acquires its characteristic flavor. Kefir grains fed with sugar water rich in minerals produce carbon dioxide as the grains consume the sugar, but not as much as in soft drinks.

When the kefir is ready, i.e. after the second fermentation, you should strain it and pour it into a jar with, say, spices, lemon, lime, pieces of fruit, ginger, or other delicious flavorings. You can put a large piece of ginger or lemon into the jar during the initial fermentation, but they will need to be removed before the mixture is strained.

WATER KEFIR FROM MILK KEFIR GRAINS

Milk kefir grains develop much faster than water kefir grains. If you make a lot of milk kefir and are left with excess milk kefir grains, you can use some of the grains to make water kefir, but note that the grains will then stop growing.

Bring 2½ cups (600 ml) of water to the boil and stir in ¼ cup (65 ml) raw sugar until it has dissolved. Cool the sugar solution to 100°F / 40°C. Mix in 2½ tbsp (35 ml) fermented milk kefir grains, cover with a cotton cloth or towel and a rubber band, and allow to ferment for three days until it has a good flavor. You will be able to use the grains for about three batches before they will need to be composted. This type of water kefir has a slightly different taste to water kefir made from water kefir grains.

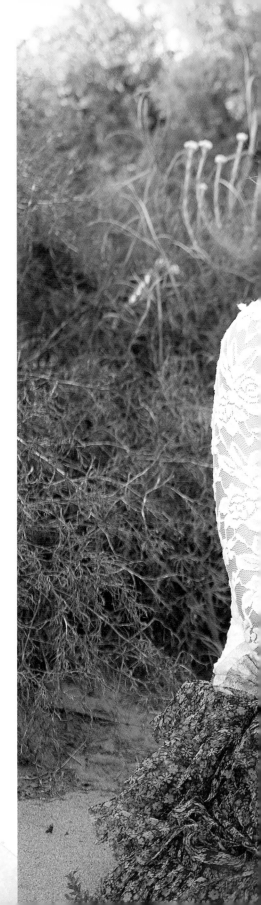

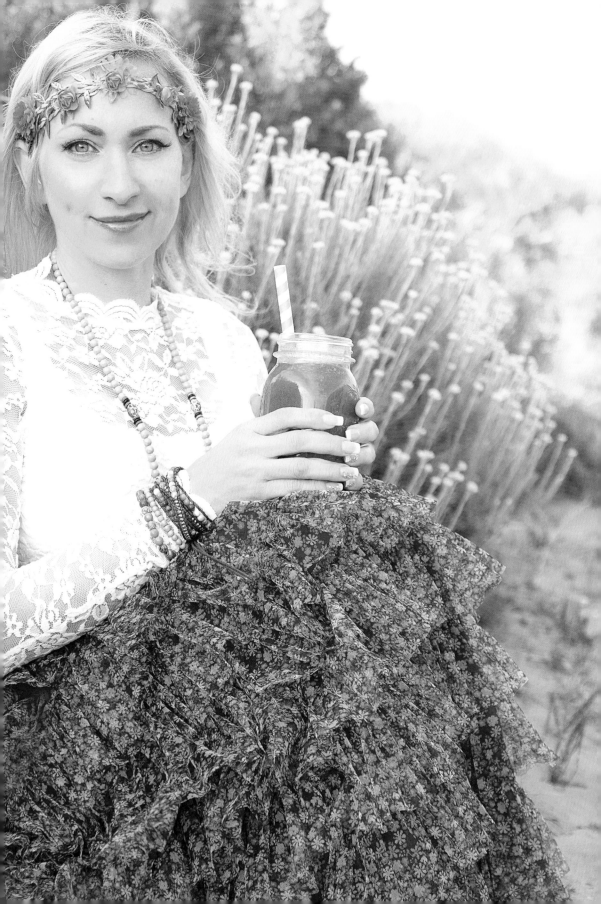

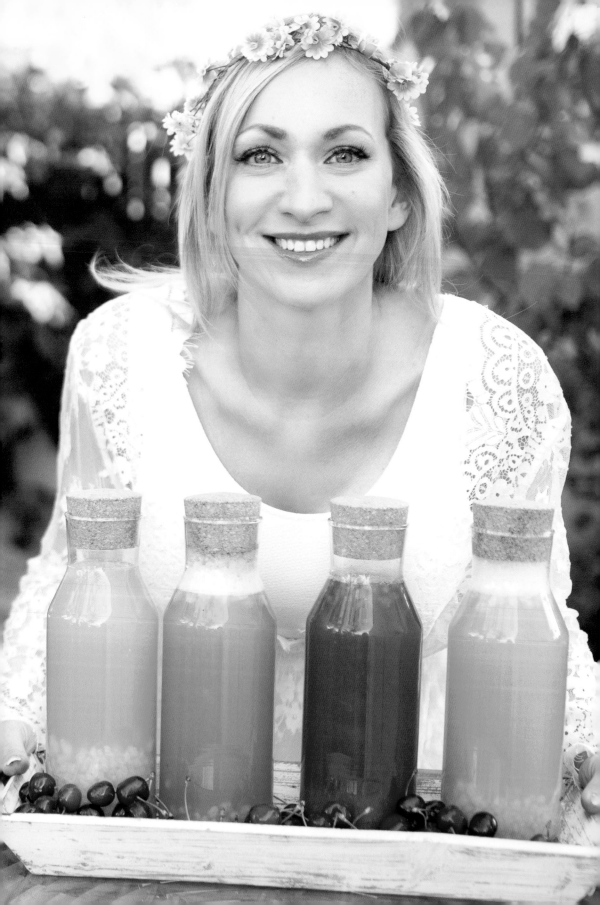

Milk kefir

THINGS YOU WILL NEED:

- ♥ 2–4 tbsp activated milk kefir grains
- ♥ 1 quart / 1 liter milk of your choice, preferably organic (not UHT), at room temperature
- ♥ a glass jar holding approx. 1½ quarts / 1.5 liters
- ♥ a towel and a rubber band
- ♥ a stainless-steel colander or nylon strainer
- ♥ if required, a cheesecloth or reusable coffee filter

1. Pour the milk into a glass jar.

2. Add the kefir grains.

3. Do not fill the jar more than three-quarters full.

4. Cover the jar with a towel and fasten with a rubber band to keep flies out.

5. Allow to stand at room temperature for between 24 and 48 hours until the milk has thickened. The exact length of time the grains should be left in the milk will depend on your personal taste, the temperature of the room, and the ratio of kefir grains to milk. The longer the milk kefir is allowed to stand, the thicker it will be. If the temperature is above 86 °F / 30 °C the process will work more quickly; in a cool room, it may take 30 to 48 hours for the milk to thicken. Do not let the kefir stand for longer than 48 hours as the grains may then start to run out of food. The kefir might also acquire laxative properties.

6. Strain the kefir to separate the grains from the liquid.

7. Store the finished drink in the fridge. It will keep for up to a week.

8. Start again from step 1.

9. If the grains have grown or increased in number, they will need more than a quart or a liter of milk, in which case it is fine to top up the jar with milk direct from the fridge.

Milk kefir can be flavored when the grains have been strained off, or, if you prefer, at the point of the second fermentation. Add fresh or dried herbs, berries, fruit, preserve, seeds, or nuts. Of course, you could also use vanilla, cinnamon, or any other spice that you like.

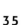

Water kefir

Just like kombucha, water kefir can be flavored with ginger, fruit, juice, herbs, spices, dried fruit, or other flavorings just as you fancy. Flavorings should be added after the kefir grains have been removed. Water kefir has a milder taste than kombucha and can be used instead of kombucha in most of the recipes in this book.

You can also make water kefir from coconut water, provided the grains have been well-established in a sugar solution beforehand. Replace the water and sugar in the recipe with a quart of coconut water and follow the instructions below.

THINGS YOU WILL NEED:

♥ 2–4 tbsp activated water kefir grains

♥ generous ¾ cup / 200 ml hot water

♥ 4 tbsp raw sugar

♥ 3⅓ cups / 800 ml cool water

♥ a glass jar holding approx. 1½ quarts / 1.5 liters

♥ a towel and a rubber band

♥ a fine-meshed nylon strainer

> **NB:**
> Honey kills bacteria and so you should not use it. If you do want to try it, you should ensure that you have enough kefir grains that it does not matter if you lose some, as the grains are unlikely to survive.

1. Heat up a generous ¾ cup / 200 ml of water. Dissolve 4 tablespoons of sugar in the water.

2. Add cold water until you have 1 quart / 1 liter of sugar solution at room temperature or cooler.

3. Add the water kefir grains to the solution.

4. Do not fill the jar more than three-quarters full.

5. Cover the jar with a towel and fasten with a rubber band to keep flies out.

6. Allow to stand at room temperature for between 24 and 48 hours. The longer the water kefir is allowed to stand, the sourer it will become. Do not allow the kefir grains to sit in the same liquid for longer than 72 hours as they may start to run out of food and then die.

7. Strain the kefir to separate the grains from the liquid.

8. Store the finished drink at room temperature or in the fridge. It will keep in the fridge for up to a week.

9. If you store the bottle at room temperature with a tight-fitting stopper, the kefir will become more carbonated.

10. Start again from step 1.

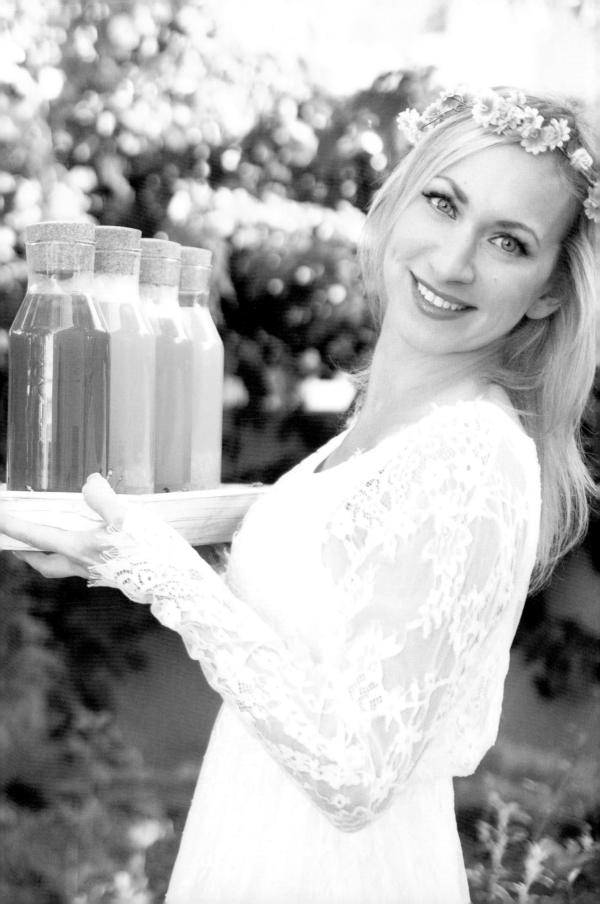

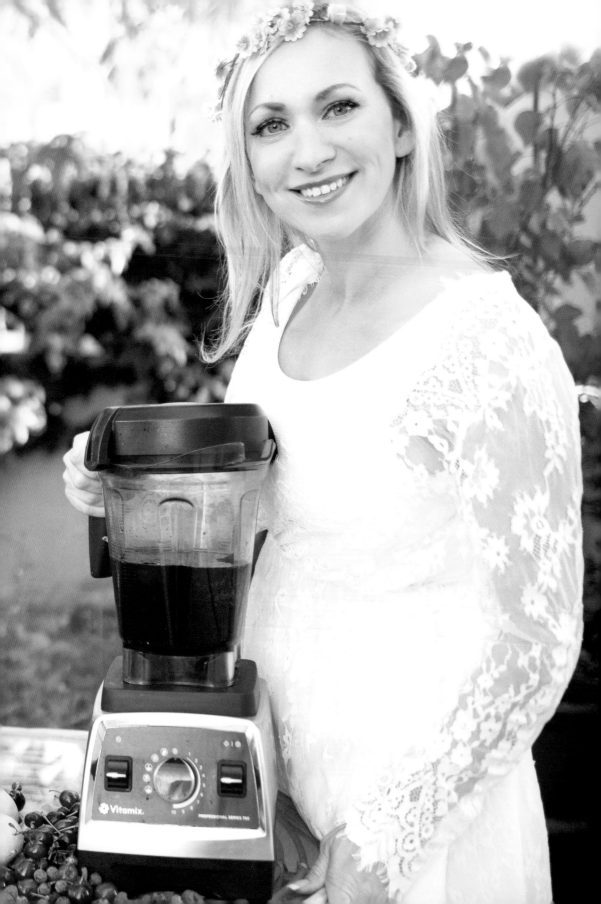

Greek kefir yogurt made from cream

If you would prefer a thicker, yogurt-like kefir rather than a drinkable version, you will find that yogurt kefir is easy to make. Try to use organic, ideally unpasteurized, cream mixed with milk. The level of fat content is up to you. You can also use just cream, but that would make it extremely rich. I like to use three quarters milk and one quarter cream for this type of kefir. You can also choose to leave out the cream, or to replace cow's milk with goat milk or another type of milk.

THINGS YOU WILL NEED:

♥ 2–4 tbsp activated milk kefir grains

♥ 3¼ cups / 750 ml milk of your choice, preferably organic (not UHT), at room temperature

♥ 1 cup / 250 ml cream, at room temperature

♥ a glass jar holding approx. 1½ quarts / 1.5 liters

♥ a towel and a rubber band

♥ a nylon strainer or stainless-steel colander

♥ if required, a cheesecloth or coffee filter

1. Pour the milk and cream into a glass jar.

2. Add the kefir grains.

3. If the grains have grown or increased in number, they will need more than a quart of the milk mixture, in which case it is fine to top up the jar with milk direct from the fridge.

4. Do not fill the jar more than three-quarters full.

5. Cover the jar with a towel and fasten with a rubber band to keep flies out.

6. Allow to stand at room temperature for 24 to 48 hours until it has thickened. The exact length of time the grains should be left in the milk will depend on your personal taste, the temperature of the room, and the ratio of kefir grains to milk. The longer the kefir yogurt is allowed to stand, the thicker it will become. If the temperature is above 86 °F / 30 °C the process will work more quickly; in a cool room, it may take 30–48 hours for the milk to thicken. Do not let the kefir stand for longer than 48 hours as the grains may then start to run out of food.

7. Strain the kefir to separate the grains from the liquid.

8. As a final step, you can strain the finished kefir through a cheesecloth or a coffee filter. That will remove a clear liquid—the whey—giving the kefir a thicker consistency, rather like curd cheese.

9. Store the finished product in the fridge. It will keep for up to a week.

10. Start again from step 1.

TIP
The whey that remains can be drunk as it is, used in smoothies, or used as a starter culture for fermenting vegetables.

Coconut kefir and yogurt

Coconut kefir and coconut kefir yogurt are almost the same. It is the fat content, i.e., the amount of coconut cream—a lot, a little, or none at all—that determines how creamy the final result is, and whether or not you strain it. The recipe below is for coconut kefir yogurt, but you can reduce the cream if you would prefer your kefir lighter.

If using coconut milk, please remember that the grains live on lactose, which coconut milk does not have. To ensure the grains do not run out of food, you must put them in regular milk after a batch or two of coconut kefir and let them rest for a few days at the top of the fridge. If you are sensitive to milk, it is important that you rinse the grains thoroughly in water at room temperature, but note that there may still be traces of milk in the coconut kefir.

THINGS YOU WILL NEED:

♥   2–4 tbsp activated milk kefir grains

♥   2 cups / 500 ml coconut milk, at room temperature

♥   2 cups / 500 ml coconut cream, at room temperature

♥   a glass jar holding approx. 1½ quarts / 1.5 liters

♥   a towel and a rubber band

♥   a stainless-steel colander or nylon strainer

♥   if required, a cheesecloth or coffee filter

TIP
The whey can be drunk as it is, used in smoothies, or used as a starter culture for fermenting vegetables.

1. Mix the coconut milk and cream until they are well blended. Transfer into a clean glass jar.

2. Add the kefir grains.

3. If the grains have grown or increased in number, they will need more than a quart or a liter of the coconut mixture, in which case it is fine to add coconut milk direct from the fridge.

4. Fill the jar up to three-quarters full.

5. Cover the jar with a towel and fasten with a rubber band to keep flies out.

6. Allow to stand at room temperature for 24 to 48 hours until thickened. The time the grains should be left in the milk will depend on your personal taste, the temperature of the room, and the ratio of kefir grains to coconut milk. The longer the kefir yogurt is allowed to stand, the thicker it will become. If the temperature is above 86 °F / 30 °C the process will work more quickly; in a cool room, it may take 30–48 hours for the milk to thicken. Do not let the kefir stand for longer than 48 hours as the grains may then start to run out of food.

7. Strain the kefir to separate the grains from the liquid.

8. As a final step, you can strain the finished kefir through a cheesecloth or a coffee filter. That will remove a clear liquid—the whey—giving the kefir a thicker consistency, rather like curd cheese.

9. Store the finished yogurt or kefir in the fridge. It will keep for up to a week.

10. Start again from step 1.

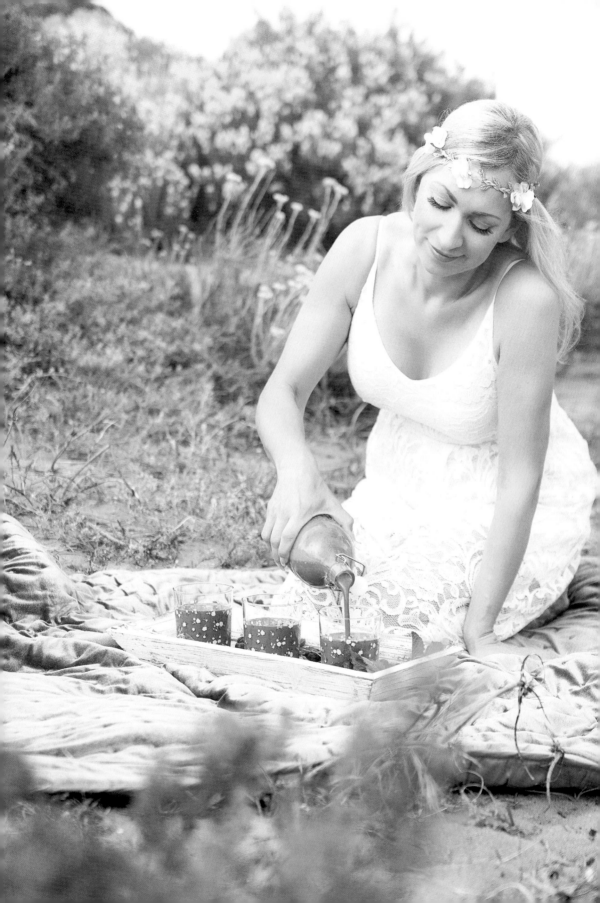

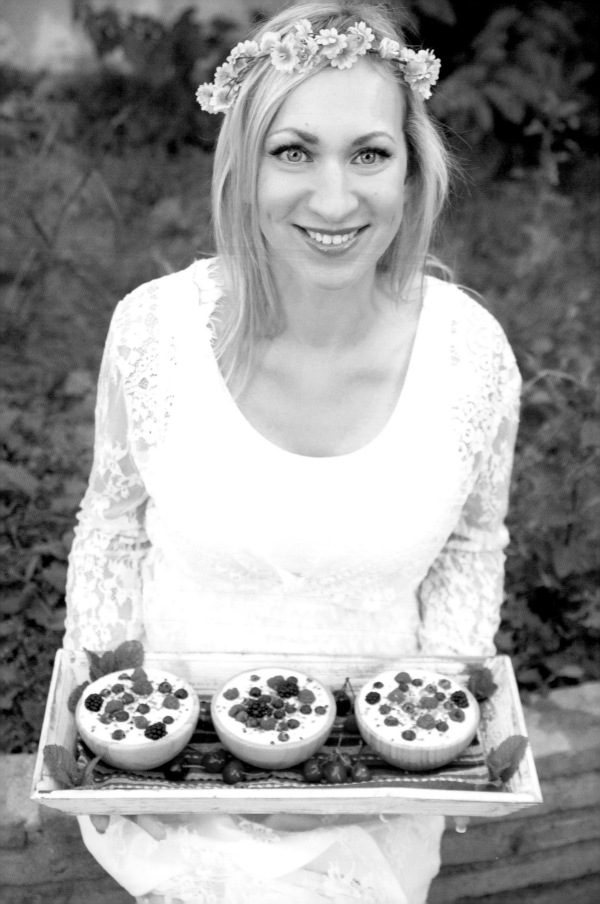

Home-made Classic Yogurt

Perhaps there was someone at home who made yogurt when you were young? Yogurt has been made at home since time immemorial, and anyone who has tasted home-made yogurt will never want to eat the store-bought variety again. Unfortunately, with higher levels of prosperity and the enormous range of products offered by stores, the tradition is increasingly disappearing.

There are two main methods for making yogurt. One uses freeze-dried yogurt culture to start the process, the other—the more common method—uses ready-made probiotic yogurt that you can buy in the stores. Obviously, you can also use a starter culture from yogurt you have made previously.

If you decide to use ready-made yogurt, choose a natural variety that you like that contains live bacteria. You will use that as a starter to ensure you get the right bacteria for your yogurt and therefore the right flavor and consistency. You only use a little starter each time you make a batch of yogurt, so the packet will last a long time. Freeze what is left over in separate small packages so that you can use them as starter at a later date. You can use any type of milk you like, but a variety with a higher fat content will work best.

THINGS YOU WILL NEED:
♥ a clean cheese or yogurt strainer
♥ a bowl with a lid
♥ 2–3 tbsp yogurt culture (normal yogurt with live bacteria or freeze-dried yogurt culture from a packet)
♥ 1 quart / 1 liter milk of your choice (not UHT—the higher the fat content the better)
♥ a saucepan
♥ a whisk
♥ 1 oz / 30 g powdered milk (optional)
♥ a 1½-quart / 1.5 liter glass jar with lid

METHOD:
1. **HEAT THE MILK.** First heat the milk to just under boiling for a few minutes. You should see small bubbles in the pan but the milk should not actually boil. The heating kills all unwanted bacteria so that the "good" bacteria gets the upper hand. If you use pasteurized, store-bought milk and clean equipment you can skip the first step.

2. **VELVETY GREEK YOGURT.** If you are making Greek yogurt, you can, if you wish, add the powdered milk and whisk it into the milk. Alternatively skip this stage.

3. **MIX IN YOUR STARTER CULTURE.** Allow the milk to cool to 104–113 °F / 40–45 °C, a little hotter than lukewarm. Pour on the starter and stir. Pour into a jar, ideally one with a lid. Do not fill the jar more than three-quarters full. One part of starter culture to nine parts of milk is usually about right in my experience.

4. **ALLOW TO STAND.** Rinse out a thermos flask with boiling water then pour in the milk mixture. The yogurt should now stand in a warm place for no less than 8 hours—up to 36 hours. The temperature should never exceed 113 °F / 45 °C, as that would kill the bacteria. You can wrap the thermos in a blanket and allow it to stand or put the yogurt into the oven at no more than 104 °F / 40 °C. If you do not have a thermos or do not want to use the oven, you can instead wrap the pan in a towel and position it somewhere warm, maximum 104 °F / 40 °C. If it is too cold, the yogurt will take longer to develop.

5. **GREEK YOGURT.** To make Greek yogurt, or just a thicker yogurt, from this, take a yogurt strainer or cheesecloth and stretch it over a bowl. Use rubber bands to keep it tight. Pour the yogurt over, place the bowl in the fridge, and allow it to strain for a few hours. The longer you leave it, the thicker the yogurt will be. Then simply remove the cloth or strainer, transfer the yogurt into a bowl with a lid and store in the fridge until you want to eat it.

6. **STORE IN A COLD PLACE.** When the yogurt has thickened, put it into the fridge for a few hours to allow it to set. This home-made yogurt is usually mild, but after a few days in the fridge it will become more acidic.

7. **SAVE THE LAST DROP.** Before you eat up the last of your yogurt, save a small amount to use as a starter for the next batch instead of store-bought yogurt. You can do that several times, but after about ten batches the yogurt will be too acidic and you will have to restart using a yogurt you have purchased as your starter culture.

TIP
The leftover whey will contain vitamins, minerals, and proteins. Do not throw it away. You can drink it as it is, add fruit and make kvass or lemonade with it, mix it into your smoothies, use it on your skin and hair, or add it to your bathwater. You can also freeze whey, and it will keep for several months.

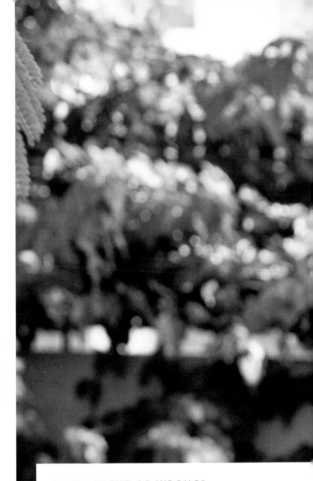

WHAT MIGHT GO WRONG?
It is difficult to fail when you are making your own yogurt. Acidity can vary from mild to really sharp, and consistency might be runny or thick, or it might separate, but this is all completely harmless. The yogurt will often not be perfect the first time round, and you will need to experiment with different temperatures and standing periods until you discover what works best for you and your yogurt. It will quickly become obvious to you if the acidification process has gone wrong. Either the yogurt will smell and taste bad or it will have gone moldy. If that happens, do not eat the yogurt, just throw it away and start again. You will need to clean (and ideally disinfect) your equipment thoroughly before using it to make yogurt again. Failure is often due to skipping step 1 or not cleaning the equipment properly.

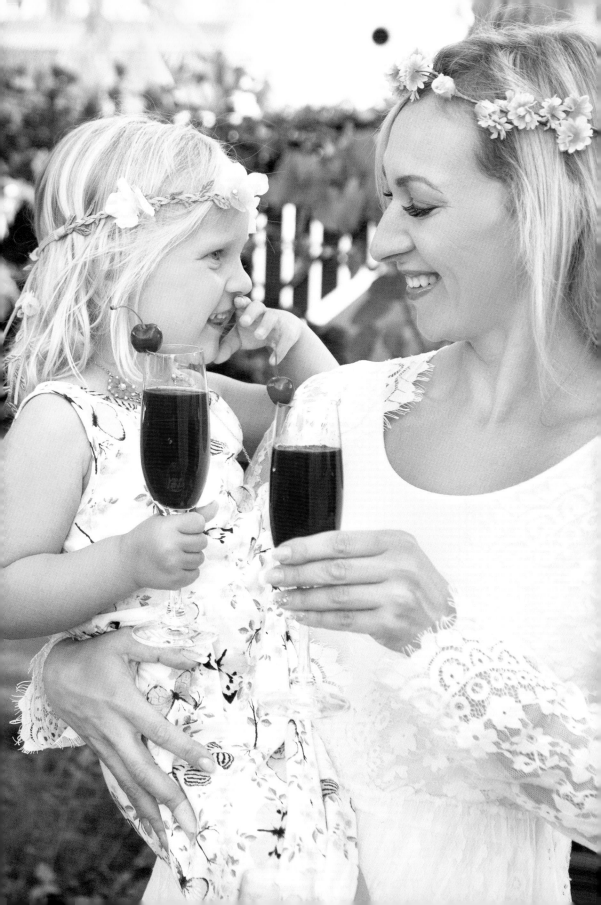

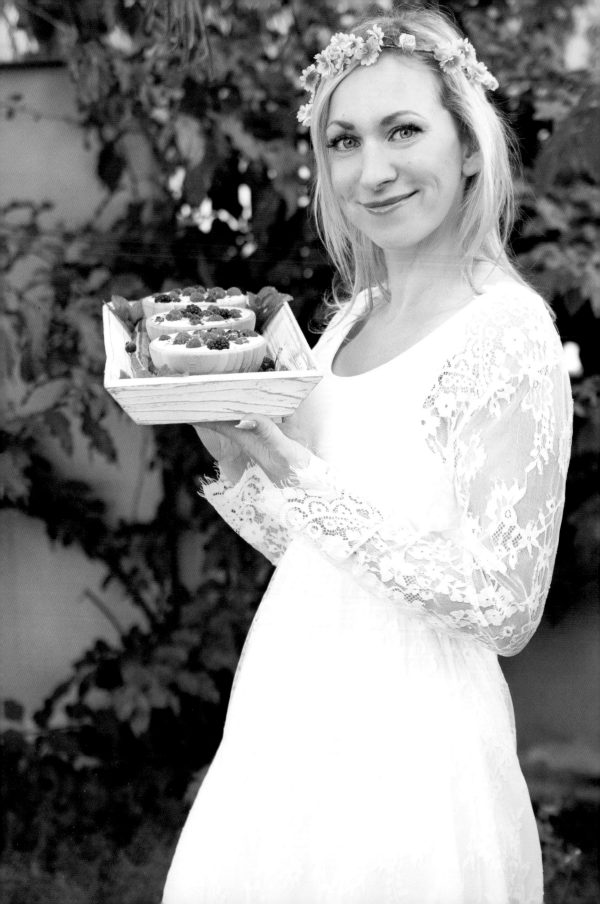

Mild Creamy Coconut Yogurt

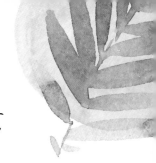

I always use additive-free organic coconut milk. For this recipe, you will also need probiotic powder or capsules. You can buy these in any health food store, in most pharmacies, and even in big food stores with a good health food section. A capsule of probiotic powder will make a generous ¾ cup / about 200 ml of coconut milk. I have tried making coconut yogurt with both kefir and kombucha, but I think the mildest version is obtained using probiotic capsules. Do some experimenting.

THINGS YOU WILL NEED:

- ♥ 2 cans (3⅓ cups / 800 ml) coconut milk, organic and additive-free
- ♥ 1 tbsp raw sugar, organic
- ♥ 4 capsules or 1½ tsp probiotic powder, starter culture
- ♥ 2 tsp tapioca (if you would like your yogurt extra thick)
- ♥ saucepan
- ♥ 1-quart / 1-liter glass jar with lid
- ♥ cotton cloth or clean towel and rubber band

1. Shake the cans of coconut milk well.

2. Heat up the coconut milk gently so that the contents are well mixed and velvety—do not boil. (You can skip heating the milk and make the yogurt from coconut milk at room temperature, but I think consistency is improved when you used heated coconut milk because the cream is mixed with the water at the bottom of the can.)

3. Add the sugar and mix well. Allow to cool, stirring all the time, until the temperature is about 104 °F / 40 °C. It must not exceed 113 °F / 45 °C, as that could kill the probiotics.

4. Split the probiotic capsules and stir the contents into the coconut milk. Add tapioca if you wish, for a thicker yogurt. Mix well.

5. Transfer into a clean glass jar. Cover with a cotton cloth or clean towel and fasten with a rubber band. This should allow the air in, but keep out flies and other undesirables.

6. You can then choose either to allow the yogurt culture to stand in a warm place (104 °F / 40 °C) overnight, so that the yogurt is ready in 10–12 hours, or let it stand for 24–48 hours at room temperature. If you choose the faster method, you can put the jar in an oven heated to 104 °F / 40 °C. Otherwise simply place the jar next to your cooker or somewhere in the kitchen that it is a little warmer. It is quite easy to tell when the yogurt is ready—it will have that delightful acidic taste. It is important that the yogurt is not in too hot a position as the heat could kill the bacteria that are needed to ferment the milk.

7. When the fermentation process is complete, put the lid on and put the jar in the fridge to chill the yogurt. It will keep happily for about a week. You can then enjoy your very own, home-made coconut yogurt. So delicious, and so very simple.

Rejuvelac

Rejuvelac is an extremely refreshing, probiotic, fermented superdrink. Just like my favorite wheatgrass shots, it derives from Ann Wigmore's theories on Living Food. Rejuvelac is traditionally made from whole, organic or biodynamically-grown wheat, which is sprouted to remove the gluten. It can also be made from other grain and seeds such as rye or barley, or from quinoa or millet for a guaranteed gluten-free alternative. It takes just under a week to make it at home, and, as with my other favorites, kombucha and kefir, no special starter culture is required.

Making your own rejuvelac is child's play. You need neither starter culture nor equipment, nor do you need many ingredients. It is also cheap. Pay strict attention to hygiene—always wash your hands before you start and use clean glass jars and cloths. In ideal conditions, the rejuvelac will be ready in five days, but if it is a little cold it can take up to just over a week.

The finished product contains protein, carbohydrates, dextrins, phosphates, saccharides, enzymes, and lactic acid bacteria. Rejuvelac is rich in enzymes and can be used as a starter culture for pickling vegetables or making your own lemonade.

THINGS YOU WILL NEED:

- ♥ 1¼ cups / 300 ml whole, organic wheat grain
- ♥ filtered water
- ♥ 1-quart / 1-liter glass jar with lid
- ♥ 3-quart / 3-liter glass jar
- ♥ glass bottles with tops

METHOD:

1. **SOAKING.** Rinse 1¼ cups / 300 ml of whole, organic wheat grain thoroughly. Soak the grain overnight or for 8–12 hours at room temperature in a lidded glass jar. Pour away the water and rinse with fresh water. Remove any damaged grain.
2. **SPROUTING.** Pour the soaked wheat grain into a large glass jar, without water. Fasten a clean cotton cloth or towel over the jar with a rubber band and place it somewhere at room temperature, for example in a kitchen cabinet. The two most important things are that the grain gets fresh air and also sits in the dark. Rinse it and drain off the water about twice a day for two days until the grain has sprouted and has small "tails".
3. **FERMENTING.** After two days, transfer the sprouts to a larger glass jar or receptacle that holds just over 3 quarts / 3 liters. Add 3 quarts / 3 liters of water. Add 3 tablespoons of honey, one tablespoon for every quart / liter of water. If you want a vegan version, replace the honey with organic raisins. This will activate the fermentation process. Cover with the cloth again. Allow to stand at room temperature for two days. If the weather is colder, the process may take up to a week.
4. **TRANSFERRING TO GLASS BOTTLES.** When the liquid turns cloudy, strain off the sprouts and pour the rejuvelac into clean glass bottles. Store the bottles in the fridge, where they will keep for about seven days. The rejuvelac may acquire a slightly sweeter flavor during this period. Drink about 1 cup / 250 ml each day to maintain good gut bacteria. Drink up to 1 quart / 1 liter a day if you have stomach problems.
5. **MAKING ANOTHER BATCH.** Do not throw the wheat away. You can reuse it to make another batch of rejuvelac. Put it back into the big jar with some fresh water. Add more honey (or fresh raisins). Allow to stand and ferment; just one day is usually enough this time round.
6. **GROWING WHEATGRASS FROM THE GRAIN.** After the second batch of rejuvelac has been made, you can sow the sprouts and grow wheatgrass, which you can then use fresh in smoothies or to make your own wheatgrass shots. If you have a lot of wheatgrass growing, you can blend it with a little water and freeze in the form of ice cubes. You will need a powerful blender for this. I grow a lot of wheatgrass, and it is really tasty and wholesome—but it took a little time to get used to the flavor.

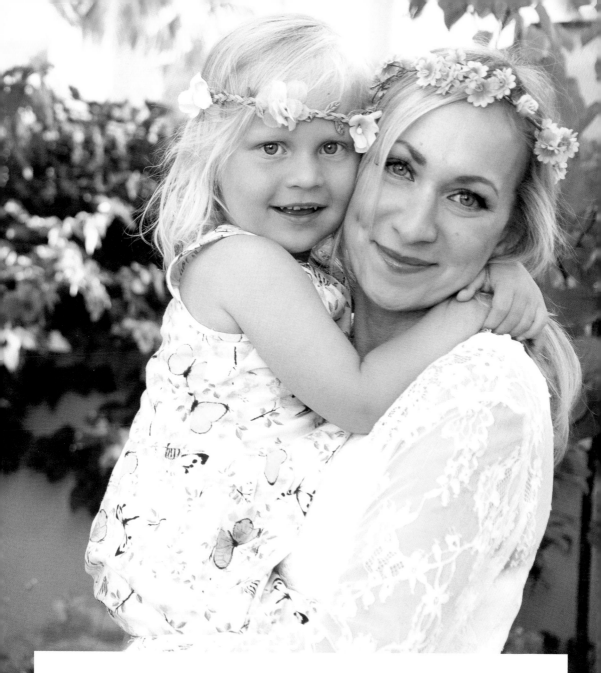

DID SOMETHING GO WRONG?

The rejuvelac should be slightly cloudy and smell and taste a bit like yogurt. If it starts to smell unpleasant and strongly acidic, it might be because you have not poured off the water during the soaking process or because there was a lid on the jar during the sprouting and fermentation stages. You may not need to throw everything away. Try rinsing the sprouts thoroughly and adding some fresh water, then start again.

DO NOT LIKE THE TASTE?

It can take a little while before you get used to it. Try mixing with a little water and squeezing some organic lemon juice or a piece of ginger into it to make it taste better. You can also use different grain—a generous ¾ cup / 200 ml of wheat and 7 tablespoons / 100 ml of rye, for example, would give a different flavor. Test some out until you find your favorite.

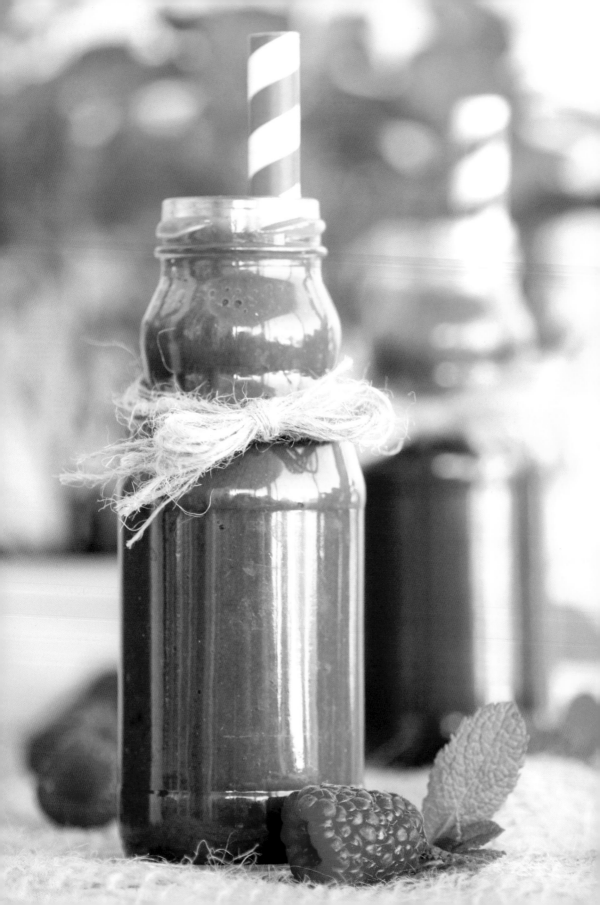

Green Kombucha Power

Kale is called *The Queen of Greens* because it has the highest vitamin content of all the vegetables from the cruciferous family (broccoli, cauliflower, white cabbage, red cabbage, and Brussels sprouts). Kale is rich in vitamins C, A, K, and B6, and also contains calcium, iron, copper, manganese, phosphorus, potassium, and several other minerals. Like all brassicas, kale promotes beneficial intestinal bacteria, cleanses the blood, and detoxifies the body. Kale is also said to contain cancer-fighting properties; it and other brassicas have been shown to limit cell growth in pancreatic cancer, and reduce the risk of cancer of the lungs, gallbladder, urinary bladder, prostate, ovaries, and rectum.

The great thing about kale is that it is available from October to March, when so many other vegetables that are grown locally and naturally are hard to come by.

MAKES 2 GLASSES

2 oz / 60 g kale, stalks removed

1 pear, cored

1 apple, cored

1 banana, frozen

1⅔ cups / 400 ml kombucha, plain

ice (optional)

Blend all the ingredients except for the ice into a smoothie. Add the ice and blend again — this makes a colder smoothie.

Gingy Pearbucha

Pears contain twice as much fiber as apples. Pears, however, do not keep as long, so make sure you buy them unripe, and store them in the fridge for a few days before using them. To speed up the ripening process, place your pears with a banana or apple in a paper bag and keep them at room temperature — bananas and apples excrete ethylene, which makes other fruits ripen faster.

I love pairing pears with ginger. Sometimes I even double or triple the ginger, but give it a try first and see what you think. You can always add more.

MAKES 2 GLASSES

3 ripe pears, cored

1–2 tsp fresh ginger, grated

1⅔ cups / 400 ml kombucha, plain

Blend all the ingredients into a great-tasting, spicy health booster.

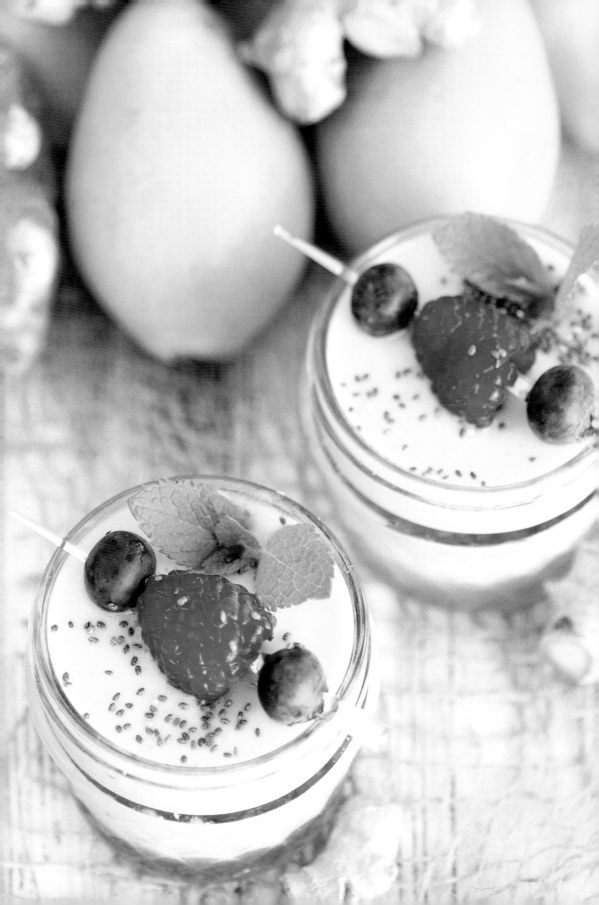

Divine Strawberry Retreat

Just 4½ ounces / 125 grams of strawberries will provide you with the full recommended daily intake of vitamin C, and a third of folate or folic acid, which is a B vitamin. Strawberries also contain a lot of fiber and minerals, such as potassium, iron, and zinc, and are high in antioxidants.

MAKES 2 GLASSES

2 tsp basil, chopped

11 oz / 300 g strawberries,
fresh or frozen

1–2 Medjool dates

1 cup / 250 ml kefir, Greek-style

ice as needed

Blend all the ingredients into a fluffy smoothie. Add the ice at the end if using fresh strawberries.

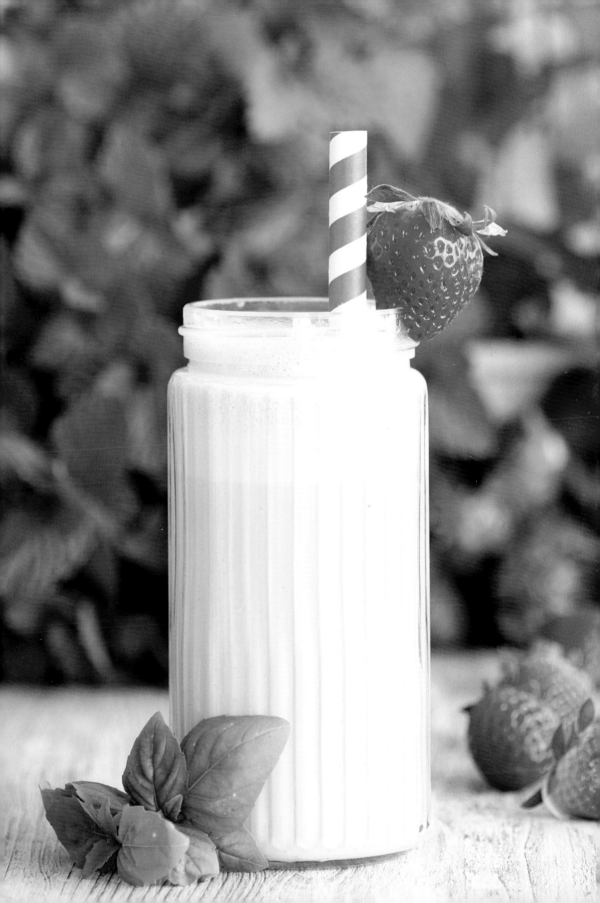

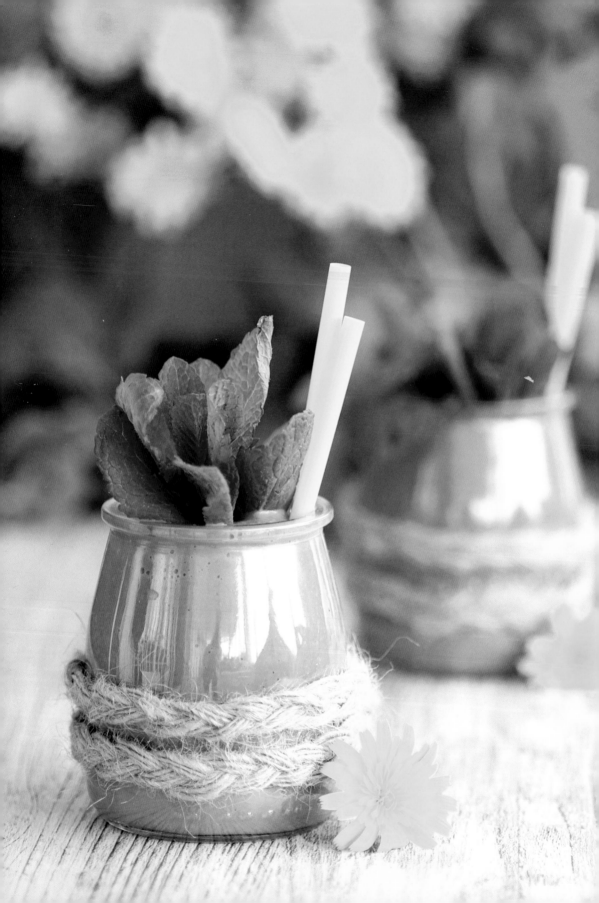

Mangolicious Love

The word "mango" comes from the Portuguese *manga*. This fruit is native to the mountainous areas of the Himalayas and Burma, and was grown in India as early as several thousand years ago. The mango tree grows to a height of 35–40 meters, and has a crown with a circumference of 8–12 meters. The flowers have a scent reminiscent of lilies. Once in bloom, it takes 3 to 6 months for the fruit to ripen. The skin varies in color, from yellow and orange to red.

When in season, you can portion mango and freeze it in plastic bags. It is much cheaper and tastier to eat frozen fruit when it is not in season than to eat fruit that has been picked unripe, stored for a long period, and sprayed with various agents to keep it fresh for months. Fresh, recently harvested fruit is always the best option, but recently harvested fruit that is immediately frozen is fine, too. To choose a flavorful mango, smell and squeeze it gently to see if it gives slightly.

TIP
If using a less powerful blender, blend the romaine and spinach with the water kefir first, then add the fruits, semi-thawed, at the end.

MAKES 2 GLASSES

3½ oz / 100 g romaine lettuce, chopped

2 oz / 60 g spinach

5½ oz / 150 g mango, frozen

3½ oz / 100 g pineapple, frozen

1⅔ cups / 400 ml water kefir

Blend all the ingredients into a divinely green smoothie.

Devilish Ginger Turmeric Kombucha

Turmeric is part of the Zingiberaceae, or the ginger family of flowering plants, and is one of the most beneficial spices around. Native to the Asian tropics, it is a perennial with a strong rhizome that contains the curcumin pigment.

Turmeric has powerful antioxidant properties against inflammation and damage caused by free radicals (residual products formed during the body's oxygenation process).

Laboratory tests have shown that turmeric may help prevent atherosclerosis, Alzheimer's disease, as well as diseases of the pancreas, liver, and lungs. Turmeric is also said to inhibit tumor growth in patients with breast, lung, skin, and prostate cancer.

If you are pregnant or trying for a baby, do not take turmeric in large quantities. Always consult your doctor if you experience any health problems.

MAKES 2 GLASSES

9 oz / 250 g mango, frozen

3½ oz / 100 g pineapple, frozen

1 tsp turmeric, grated (or ½ tsp ground turmeric)

1–2 tsp ginger, grated

1⅔ cups / 400 ml kombucha, plain

Blend all the ingredients into a golden smoothie.

TIP
If using a less powerful blender, allow the frozen fruit to thaw before blending, or use fresh fruit.

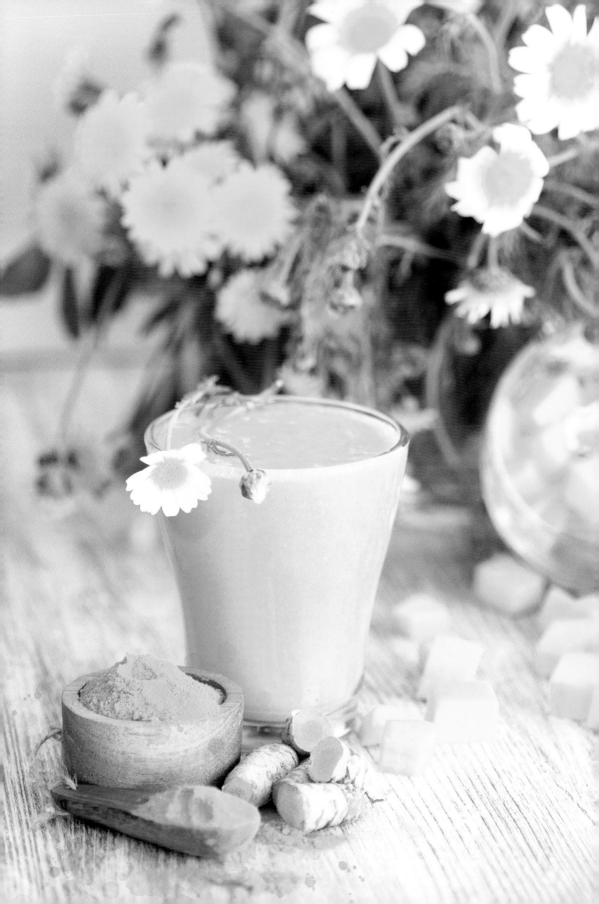

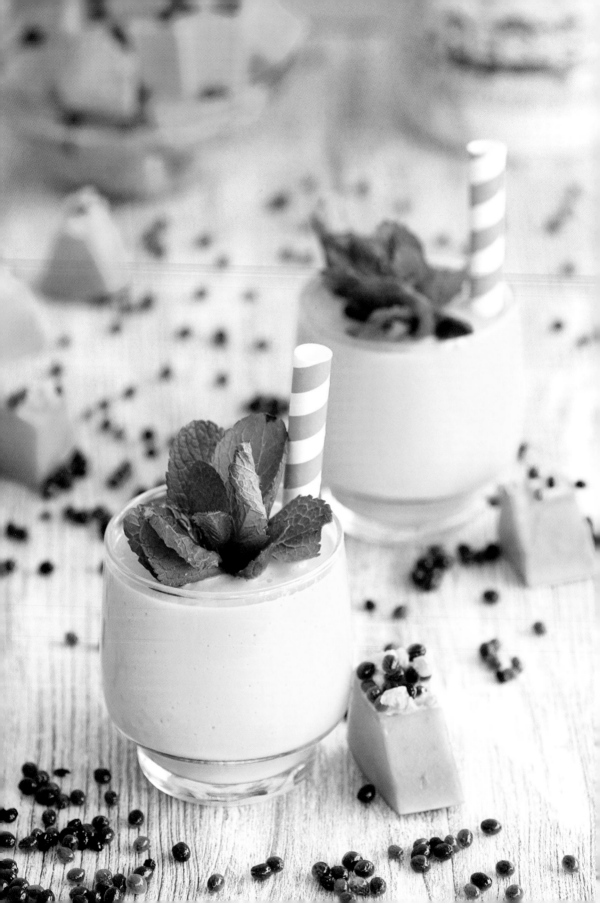

Papaya Passion

Papaya is rich in vitamins A, C, E, and B, as well as many antioxidants, such as carotene, zeaxanthin, and flavonoids. It also contains many important minerals, such as potassium, magnesium, calcium, and iron. Papaya contains the enzyme papain, which is used as a medicine against digestive problems. Papaya is also said to be effective for weight loss.

MAKES 2 GLASSES

9 oz / 250 g papaya, frozen

3½ oz / 100 g pineapple, frozen

1 tsp chia seeds

1 cup / 250 ml kombucha, plain

Blend all the ingredients into a yummy smoothie.

TIP
If using a less powerful blender, allow the fruit to thaw before blending, or use fresh fruit.

Dandelion Dream

Dandelion sap contains a number of bitter substances that stimulate the appetite and increase the flow of saliva and glandular secretions in the gastrointestinal tract and the liver. In late summer, it is the root that has the highest content of these substances; in the spring, it is the leaves. In addition to the bitter substances, the leaves contain B and C vitamins and potassium. Dandelions have a strong diuretic effect. In Germany and Austria, dandelions are prescribed for gall bladder and liver disorders and for gout and rheumatism.

Dandelions can be made into wine or syrup, form the basis of a tasty salad, or be brewed into a tea. During the 1940s war years, the root used to be roasted and used as a coffee substitute. A 14-day course of treatment with fresh dandelion stalks is said to cure fatigue and weakness. The plant is also said to purify the blood and act as a tonic.

MAKES 2 GLASSES

1 oz / 30 g dandelion leaves

1 oz / 30 g alfalfa sprouts (or other mild sprouts)

11 oz / 300 g honeydew melon

juice of ½ lemon

1–2 dates

1 cup / 250 ml water kefir

Blend all the ingredients into a green smoothie.

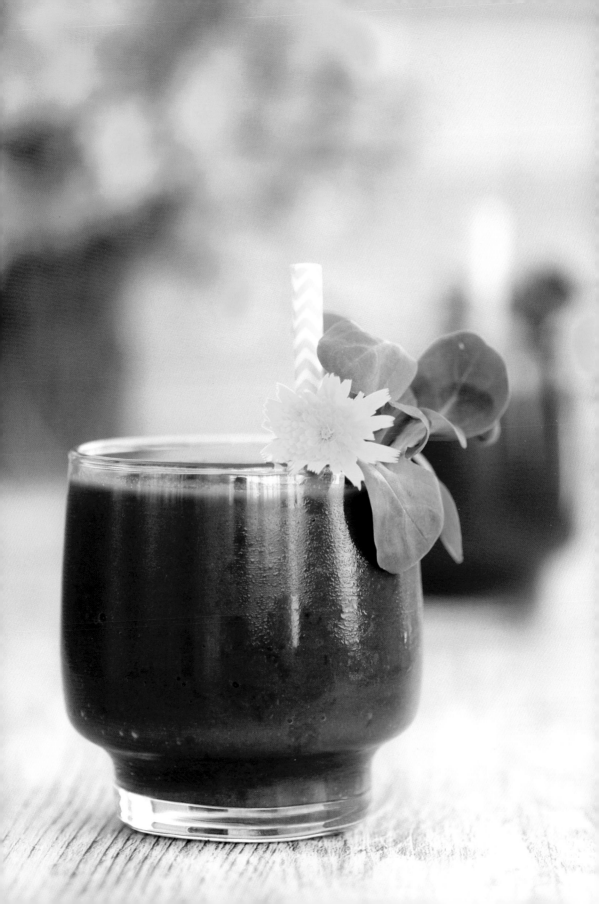

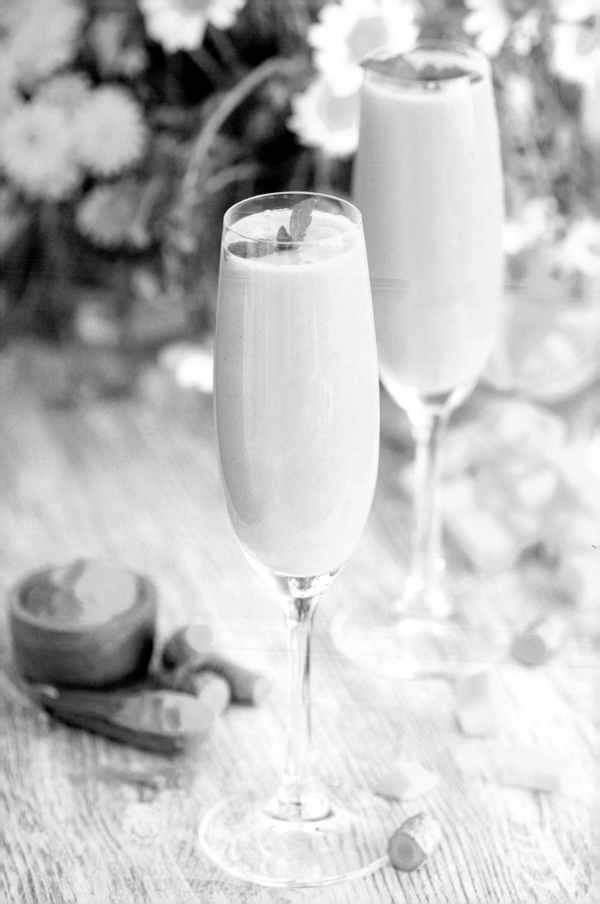

Liquid Gold

Fresh turmeric can be grown in the same way as ginger. Plant the root in a plant pot in early spring. It can stand outdoors in the summer and be harvested in the autumn. If the root is hard to grate, try freezing it and grating it when frozen. If you rinse and scrub the skin thoroughly, it will not need peeling. Be careful when handling fresh turmeric, as it can seriously stain your hands and your kitchen, and is very difficult to remove. Use gloves or hold it with a small plastic bag.

Because piperine, the active ingredient of black pepper, has been found to substantially increase the absorption of curcumin, the active ingredient of turmeric, I recommend that you use a mix of the two.

MAKES 2 GLASSES

5½ oz / 150 g mango, frozen

juice of 2 oranges

1–2 tsp turmeric, grated (or ½–1 tsp ground)

1 tsp cinnamon, ground

pinch black pepper

1 cup / 250 ml kombucha, plain

Squeeze the oranges. Blend all the ingredients into a golden-yellow smoothie.

Radical Beet Detox

Red beets contain calcium, vitamin C, iron, magnesium, phosphorus, and manganese among other nutrients. They are said to cleanse the blood and promote red blood cell growth. Studies have shown that red beets increase the body's capacity to take up oxygen and improve stamina during exercise. Beets are also considered to be helpful for high blood pressure and ulcers and are also believed to remove toxins from the intestines, liver, and gallbladder.

MAKES 2 GLASSES

2 oz / 60 g romaine lettuce, chopped

5½ oz / 150 g red beets, peeled and chopped
(fresh or pre-cooked)

2 apples, cored

1–2 tsp ginger, grated

1⅔ cups / 400 ml kombucha, plain

ice as needed

Blend all the ingredients into a deep red, purifying
health elixir. For a colder smoothie, blend in some
ice at the end.

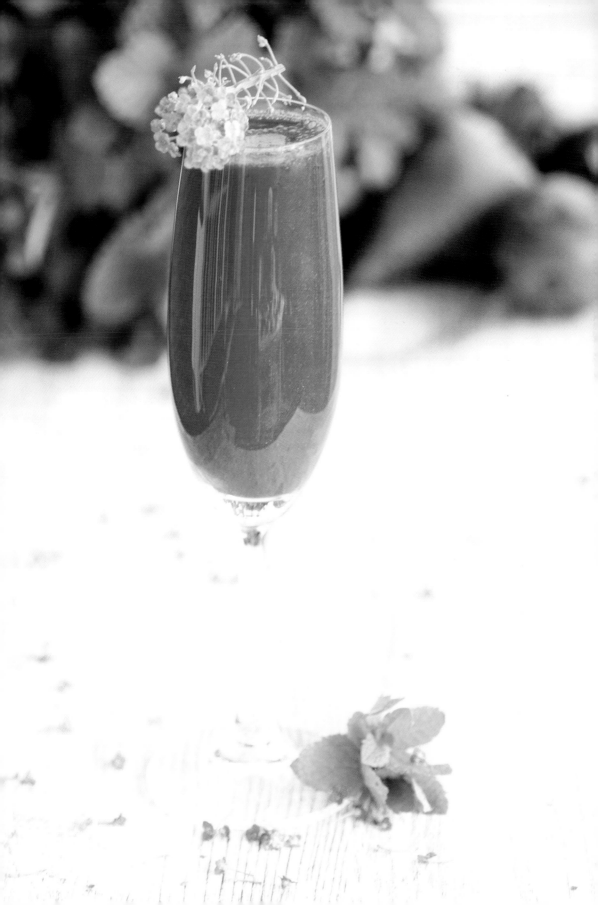

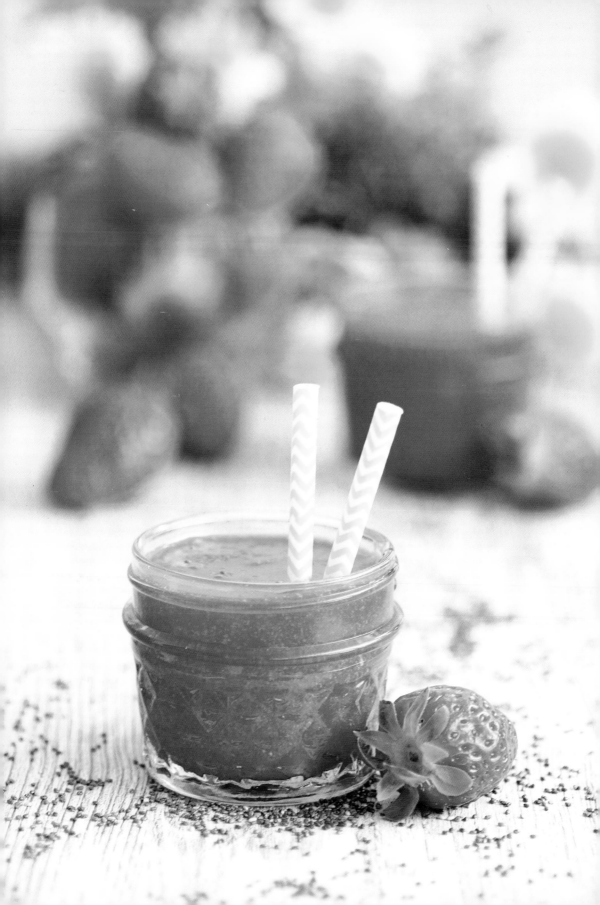

Jungle Strawberry Fever

Coconut water has become extremely popular, both as a restorative after a hard work-out and as a useful addition to smoothies. Coconut water is the clear liquid found in young, green coconuts. It is 95 percent water, the remainder consisting of nutrients and minerals such as vitamin B, vitamin C, phosphorus, calcium, and zinc. Sometimes called "nature's own sports drink," it is particularly rich in potassium.

Coconut water should not be confused with coconut milk, which is produced from the white flesh of ripe, brown coconuts. Coconut water freezes very nicely in ice-cube trays and will keep for six months in your freezer.

MAKES 2 GLASSES

7 oz / 200 g strawberries

7 oz / 200 g pineapple, frozen

1 cup / 250 ml coconut water

1 cup / 250 ml kombucha, plain

Blend all the ingredients into a smooth consistency.

Energizing Spicy Green Fuel

Chai is an Indian spice mix that is normally consumed as tea. The mixture can consist of many different spices, but usually contains cardamom, cinnamon, and ginger. Chai is almost always served with milk, and is sometimes even boiled in milk for a more intense flavor.

It is easy to make your own chai mix and then store it in an airtight container in a cool place: 2 tsp cardamom, 2 tsp cinnamon, 1 tsp nutmeg, 1 tsp cloves, 1 tsp ginger, and 1 tsp black pepper. The more freshly ground the spices, the more intense their flavor and fragrance. I always grind all my own spices in a coffee grinder.

MAKES 2 GLASSES

2 apples (Granny Smith)

2 oz / 60 g spinach

1–2 tsp chai spice mix

1–2 dates, pitted

1⅔ cups / 400 ml kombucha

ice

Blend all the ingredients into a smoothie. For a colder smoothie, add some ice at the end.

TIP
If you are using a less powerful blender or non-organic apples, peel the apples first.

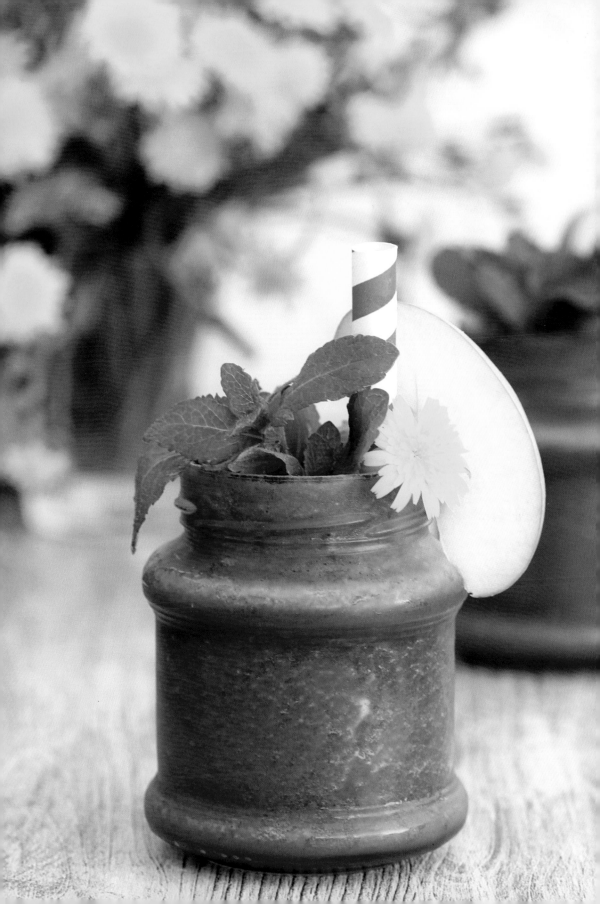

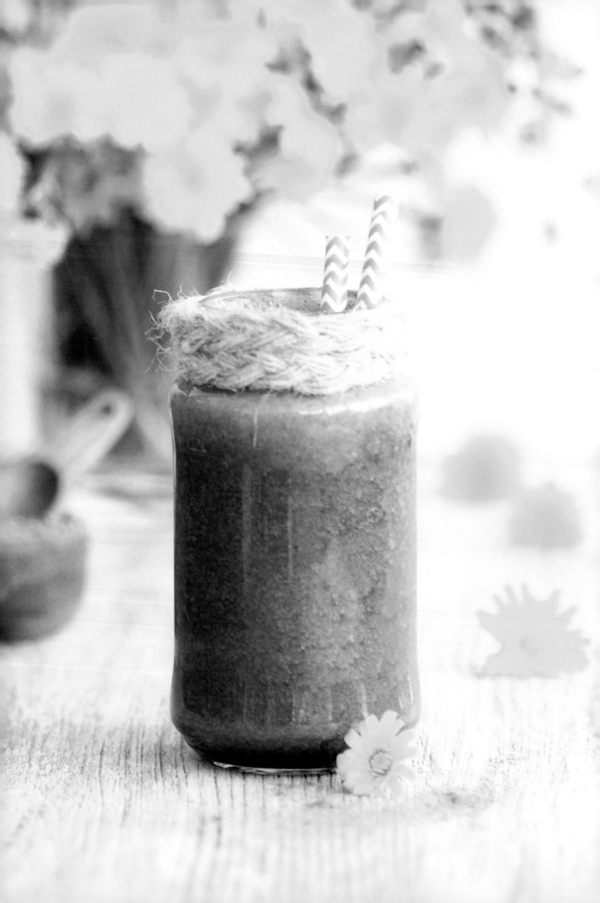

Happy Grasshopper

Pineapple is a deliciously sweet fruit that contains large amounts of beneficial dietary fiber and vitamins that provide protection against viruses and infections. It is particularly rich in vitamin C, which builds up connective tissue and helps the body absorb iron from food. Vitamin C is also an antioxidant that protects against free radicals, which have damaging effects on the body's cells. In addition to vitamins, pineapple is also rich in bromelain, a powerful enzyme that breaks down proteins and thereby aids digestion. Bromelain is also said to be good for the circulation and able to lower blood pressure.

When buying a pineapple, look for one that is plump. To check whether it is ripe, try carefully pulling off one of the lower leaves. If it comes off, the pineapple is ripe. But it could also be over-ripe, so it is best to choose one whose leaves do not come off and allow it to ripen at home.

When in season, I rinse pineapples, cut off the top, skin and tough core, cut the flesh into pieces that I freeze on a baking tray covered with parchment paper. Once the pineapple has frozen, I transfer the frozen pieces to a re-sealable plastic bag and mark with contents and date. They will keep in the freezer for up to six months.

MAKES 2 GLASSES

9 oz / 250 g pineapple, frozen

1–2 tsp ginger, grated

2–3 tsp wheatgrass powder (or a handful of fresh)

1⅔ cups / 400 ml water kefir

Blend all the ingredients into a yummy health boost.

Tibetan Delight

Goji berries and their health benefits have been known to the Chinese for over 5,000 years, but in Europe their major breakthrough came at the start of the 21st century. Nowadays you can buy goji berries anywhere. I always buy organic goji berries. One of my favorite goji berry producers actually comes from Tibet.

Goji berries have proved to be one of the most nutritious foods there is. Uniquely, they contain, amongst other things, 18 different amino acids, of which seven are essential to life. They are also packed with important minerals such as iron, calcium, zinc, selenium, copper, potassium, germanium, and phosphorus. They are also rich in vitamins B1, B2, B6, and E.

MAKES 2 GLASSES

3 tbsp goji berries

1 cup / 250 ml kombucha

9 oz / 250 g mango, frozen

1 tsp turmeric, grated
(or ½ tsp ground)

Soak the goji berries in the kombucha for 10–15 minutes; I usually soak them direct in the blender jar. Blend all the ingredients into a wonderfully orange vitamin C boost.

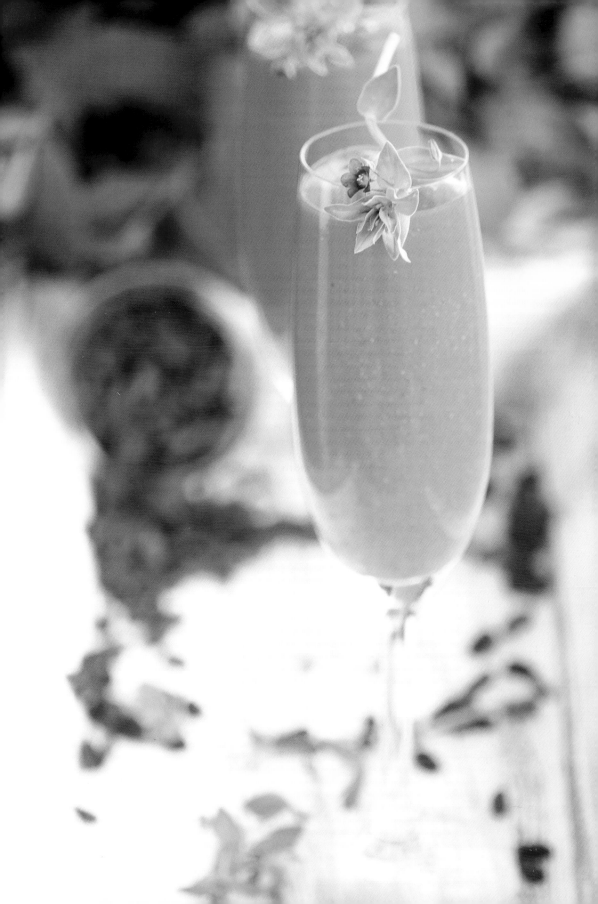

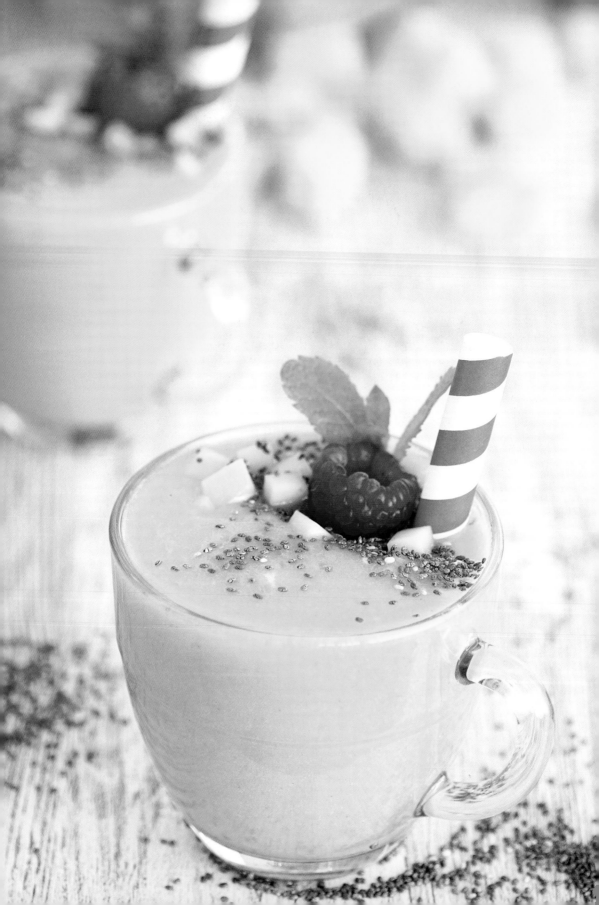

Californian Sunshine

Most people know that oranges contain a lot of vitamin C, but they may not be aware that they also contain other healthy substances that you canot get from an effervescent tablet. In addition to strengthening the immune system, lowering blood pressure, and preventing colds and infections, oranges are said to provide extra protection against eye diseases, rheumatism, cardiovascular disease, and cancer. The vitamin C in the orange is also revitalizing for the skin.

Vitamin C enhances the body's take-up of several nutrients, including iron, zinc, copper, calcium, and vitamin B9 (folic acid). It also has an antioxidant effect on other substances in the body and helps to break down damaging free radicals. Vitamin C cannot be stored in the body and so the body must take in fresh supplies every day.

MAKES 2 GLASSES

2 tsp chia seeds

1 cup / 250 ml kombucha, plain

2 oranges, peeled

juice of 2 grapefruit

3½ oz / 100 g mango, frozen

3½ oz / 100 g pineapple, frozen

Soak the chia seeds in the kombucha for 10–15 minutes. Blend all the ingredients into a smooth consistency.

Fountain of Youth

Aloe barbadensis counts as one of our oldest known medicinal plants. It has been used in traditional medicine across the world for thousands of years. Today, aloe vera features as an ingredient in many different drinks and concentrated juices but not always in large quantities, so always read the label so you can see what the aloe vera content is. Aloe vera juice should contain pure, concentrated, cold-pressed juice from cultivated *Aloe barbadensis* plants.

As the Swedish proverb says, "A beloved child has many names." Aloe vera is also called gift of Venus, the medicine plant, the potted physician, the miracle plant, heaven's magic wand, or the burn plant.

Fresh aloe vera can have a laxative effect in large doses, so keep your intake low.

MAKES 2 GLASSES

1 oz / 30 g spinach

½ avocado

5½ oz / 150 g pineapple, frozen

⅔ cup / 150 ml aloe vera juice

1 cup / 250 ml rejuvelac

2 tsp wheatgrass powder (or a handful of fresh)

Blend all the ingredients into a smooth consistency.

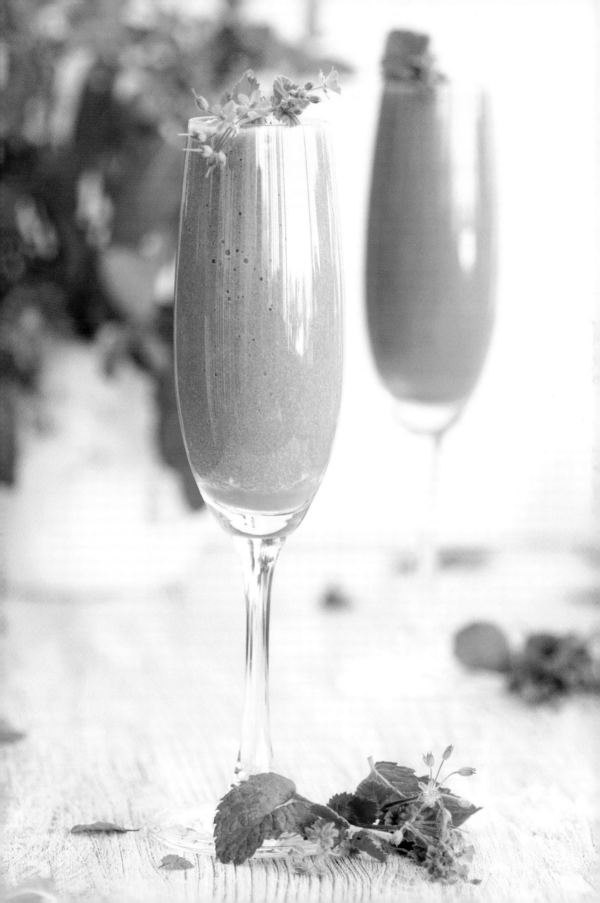

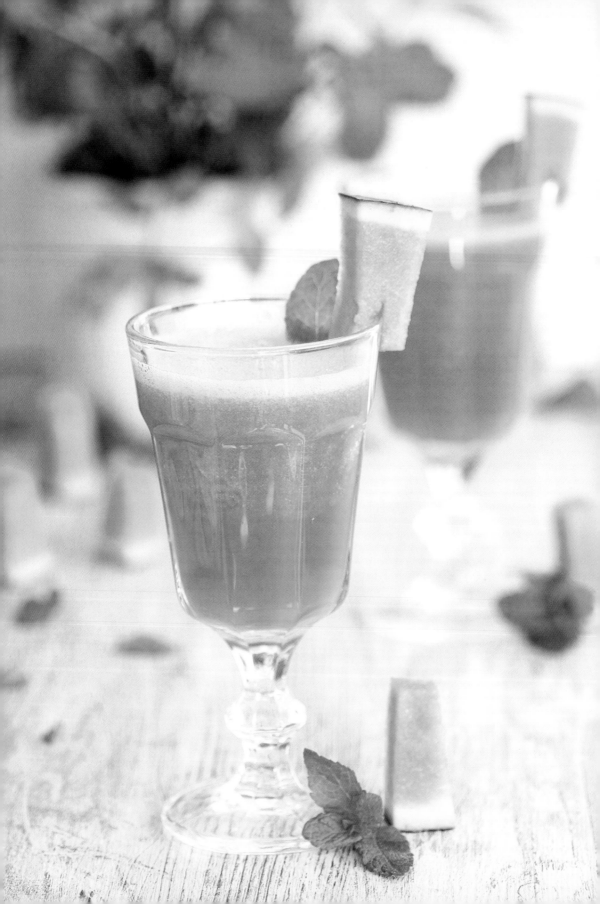

Hot Watermelon

Watermelon is one of the few foods to contain generous amounts of the powerful antioxidant lycopene, which is said to reduce the risk of heart disease and certain types of cancer, such as cervical cancer and prostate cancer. It is also a good source of vitamins A, C, and B6.

There are many different types of watermelon. Most have dark pink or red flesh, but some varieties have a golden hue. They can be round or oblong in shape, and weigh between 4½ and 44 lb (or between 2 and 22 kg). Most have a roughly similar taste, but the level of sweetness can vary greatly. I like to use large, oblong, red-fleshed watermelons.

Avoid melons that are split or marked. The skin should be firm, matt, and butter-yellow on the underside where the melon has ripened against the ground. Ripe watermelons have a slight scent and should feel quite heavy—they are 92 percent water.

MAKES 2 GLASSES

2 tsp chia seeds

1⅔ cups / 400 ml water kefir

14 oz / 400 g watermelon, cubed

¼– ½ chili

juice of ½ lime

Soak the chia seeds in the water kefir for 10–15 minutes. Blend all the ingredients into a smooth consistency.

Maqui Blueberry-bucha

Maqui berries originate from Patagonia in southern Chile. They rank high on the ORAC list, which compares the antioxidant values of different foods. Maqui berries have four times the antioxidants of blueberries and twice as much as açaí berries. That makes maqui berries an effective weapon against free radicals. They are also said to protect the body's cells against oxidative stress and counteract premature aging. The antioxidants strengthen the immune system, help reduce inflammation, and stabilize blood sugar levels. Maqui berries are also bursting with flavonoids, polyphenols, vitamins A, C, and E, and the minerals calcium, iron, and potassium.

MAKES 2 GLASSES

1 banana, frozen

9 oz / 250 g blueberries, wild

2 tbsp maple syrup (grade B)

1 tsp cinnamon, ground

2 tsp maqui berry powder

1⅔ cups / 400 ml kefir, Greek-style

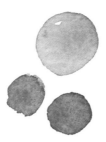

Blend all the ingredients into a smooth consistency.

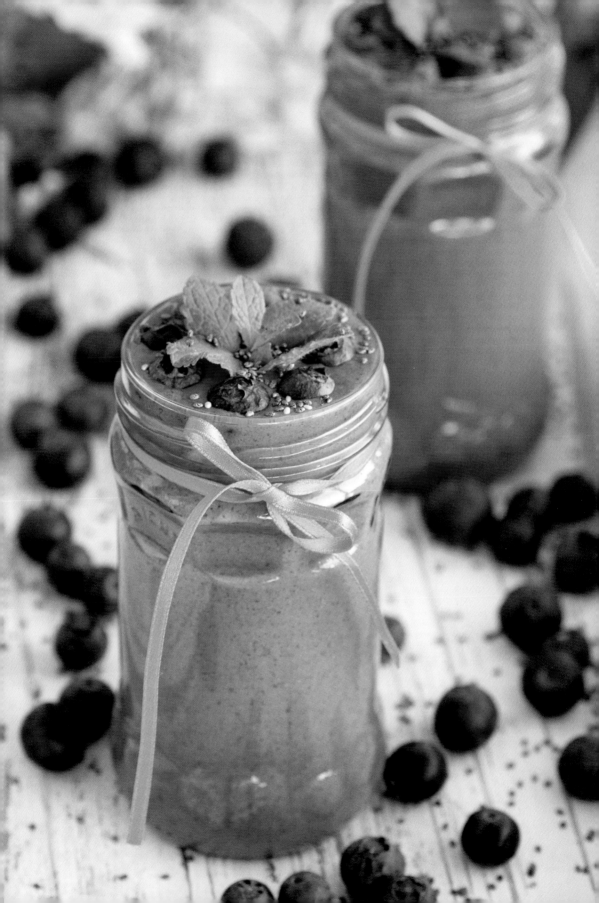

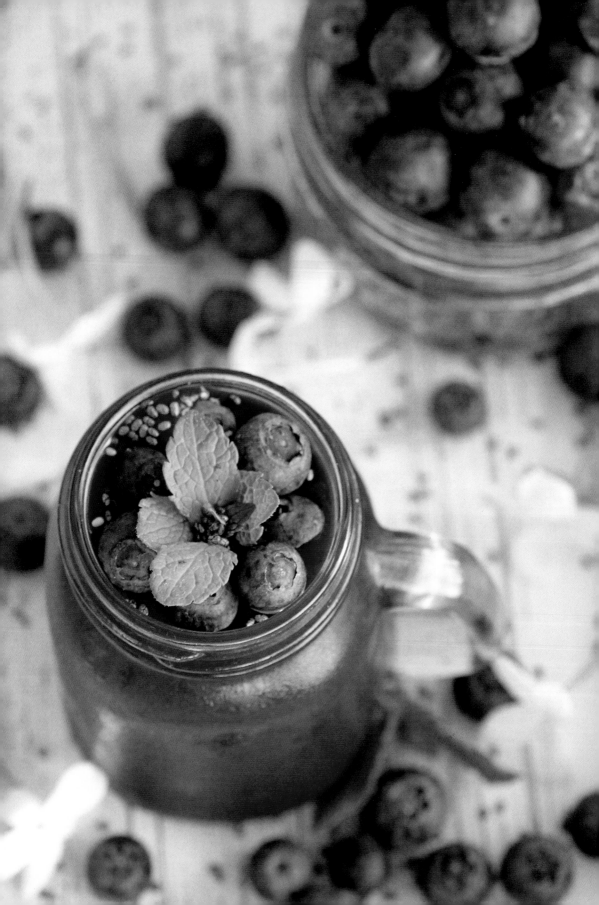

Brain Power Fuel

Ginkgo biloba is one of the world's best-selling herbal medicines. The herb, also known as the Chinese temple tree, is said to improve circulation, help counter a poor memory, enhance powers of concentration, and protect against dementia.

TIP
The tea will keep in a clean, sealed glass bottle for up to a week.

MAKES 2 GLASSES

1 cup / 250 ml ginkgo biloba tea, cooled

⅔ cup / 150 ml kombucha, plain

2 tsp chia seeds

9 oz / 250 g blueberries, frozen

½ tsp cinnamon, ground

¼ tsp cardamom

½ tsp ginger, grated

pinch cayenne pepper

Make the tea according to the instructions on the packet and allow it to cool. Soak the chia seeds in either the kombucha or the tea for 10–15 minutes. Blend all the ingredients into a delicious, blueish-purple health drink.

Strawberrita

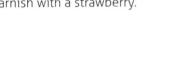

A delicious, non-alcoholic summer drink that makes a good aperitif at parties. Yum. And it is healthy too.

MAKES 2 GLASSES

11 oz / 300 g strawberries, frozen

½ tsp vanilla powder or extract

zest of ½ lime

2 tbsp coconut nectar sugar or maple syrup (grade B)

1⅔ cups / 400 ml kombucha

Blend all the ingredients into a wonderfully red, tempting summer drink. Garnish with a strawberry.

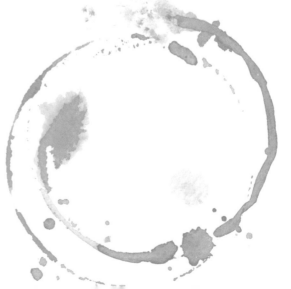

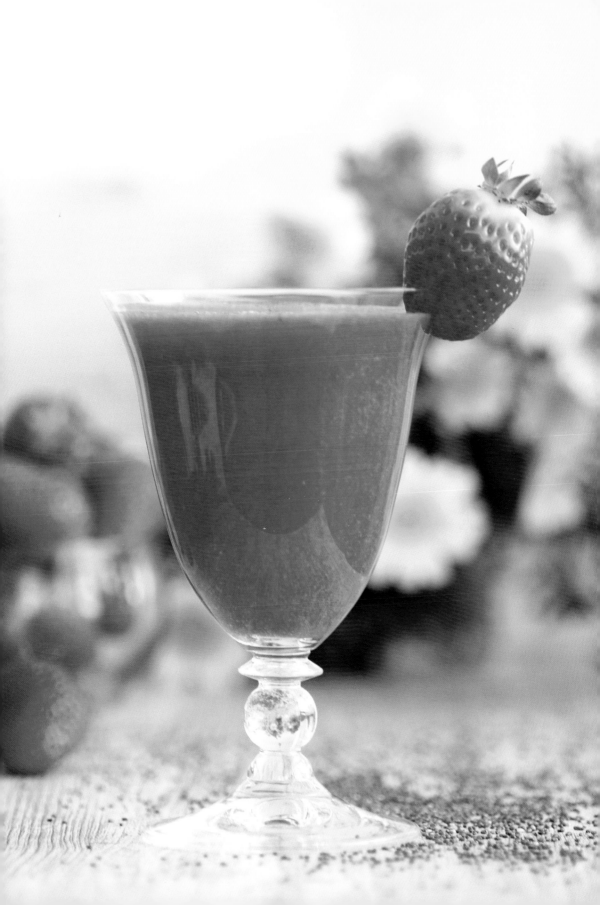

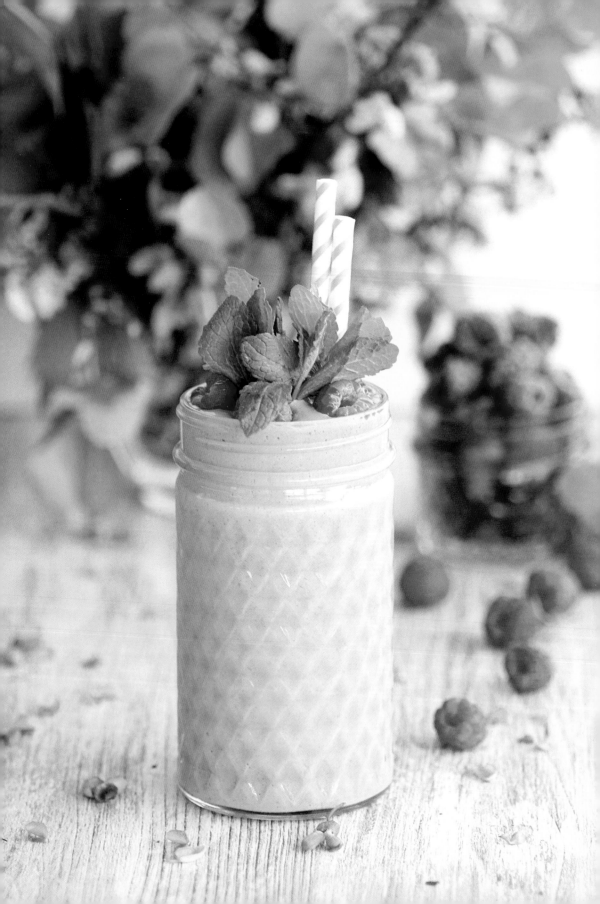

Double Probiotic Potion

Banana is the perfect sweetener for smoothies. I usually buy large quantities of organic bananas when slightly spotted, almost over-ripe bananas are available at a good price. They are good for freezing, having a pleasant sweetness and creamy consistency. Peel and slice the bananas into small pieces and freeze on a baking sheet covered with parchment paper. When they are well frozen, transfer into a re-sealable plastic bag. They will keep for up to six months. Don't forget to write the contents and date on the bag.

MAKES 2 GLASSES

2 tsp chia seeds

⅔ cup / 150 ml kombucha, plain

5½ oz / 150 g raspberries

5½ oz / 150 g strawberries

1 banana, frozen

1¼ cups / 300 ml kefir, Greek-style

1–2 Medjool dates, pitted

ice as needed

Soak the chia seeds in the kombucha for 10–15 minutes. Blend all the ingredients into a wonderfully smooth, dreamy pink smoothie. Add some ice cubes at the end to taste.

Pina Colada-bucha

A classic Caribbean drink with a twist—non-alcoholic and healthy.

When coconuts are allowed to ripen, the coconut water becomes thick and milk-like—this is real coconut milk. The coconut milk that can be bought in cans in food stores is often coconut extract blended with water. Most cans are labeled so that you can see how much of the contents comes from coconut and how much is added water. Always buy unsweetened, additive-free coconut milk.

Coconut milk is a delicious and creamy alternative to milk and cream when you are cooking, and is also completely lactose-free. Fat content varies, but is usually around 25 percent. Coconut milk contains large amounts of minerals such as potassium, iron, magnesium, and phosphorus.

You can make small amounts of coconut milk yourself by blending grated coconut with water and then draining off the flesh. Coconut milk works well frozen in ice-cube trays.

MAKES 2 GLASSES

⅔ cup / 150 ml coconut milk

⅔ cup / 150 ml kombucha, plain

9 oz / 250 g pineapple, frozen

1 tsp vanilla powder or extract

Blend all the ingredients into a creamy smoothie and enjoy.

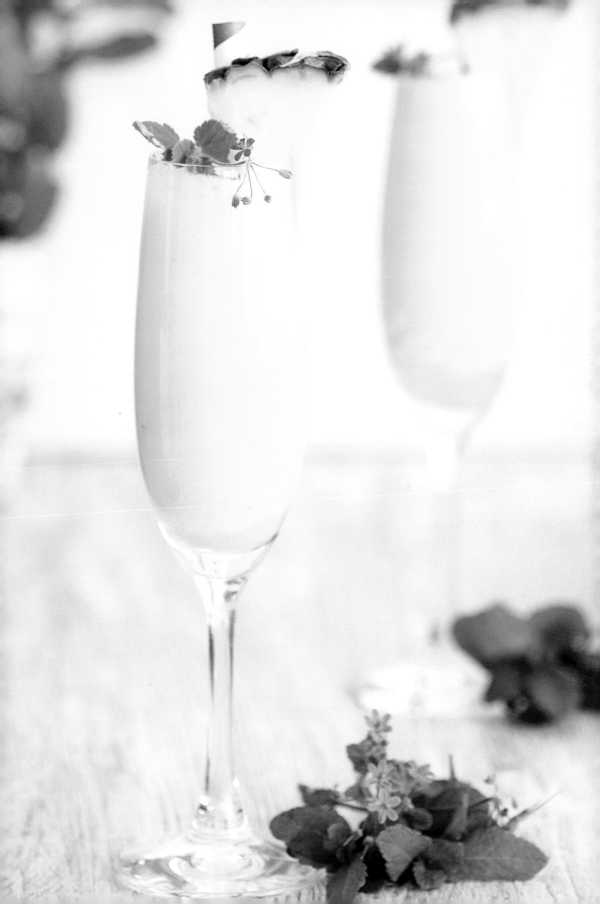

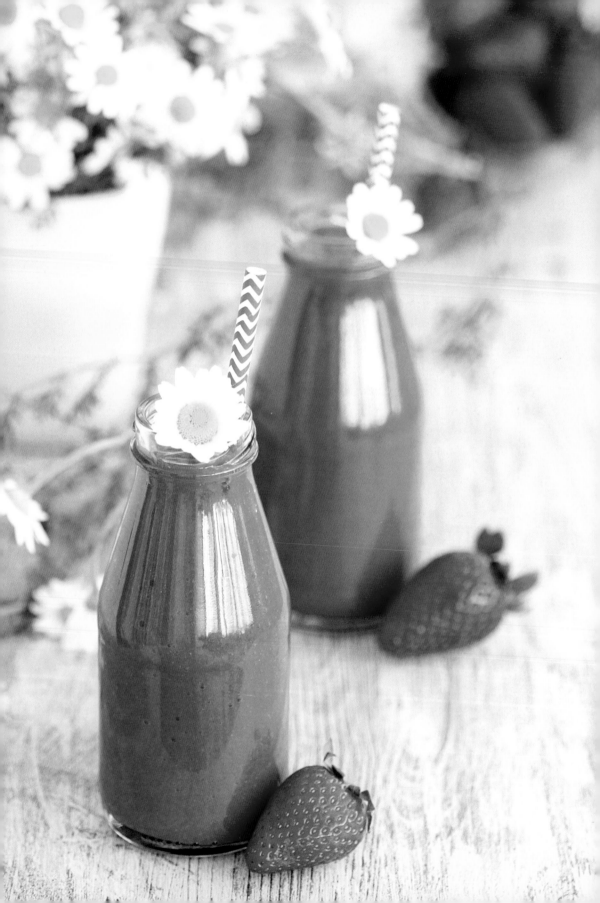

Flower Power

Chamomile is one of the oldest and most popular medicinal plants in Europe. It grows wild in fields and on verges across the whole continent, and is gathered mainly for the healing properties of its daisy-like flowers. Chamomile contains several active medicinal substances and essential oils, such as the blue colorant chamazulene. Chamomile can be used both externally and internally as an anti-inflammatory and an anti-bacterial agent, and also as a sudorific. It is also said to have a calming and soothing effect.

Dried or fresh chamomile flowers are normally used to make tea; one to two teaspoonfuls of dried herbs for each large cup, depending on the required strength. The tea is good for stomach and intestinal ailments, gastritis, and colicky pains. A couple of cups can help with menstrual pain. Chamomile tea can also soothe tension headaches and minor migraines and is thought to have both a preventive and healing effect on colds. If you have difficulty relaxing in the evening, a cup of chamomile tea will calm you.

You should not use chamomile if you are allergic to composite flowers.

MAKES 2 GLASSES

1 cup / 250 ml chamomile, marigold, or lavender tea, cooled (or a mixture of all three)

6–8 apricots, pitted

3½ oz / 100 g raspberries

3½ oz / 100 g strawberries

1–2 tsp bee pollen

1 cup / 250 ml kombucha, plain

Make the tea—use 2 teaspoonfuls of chamomile, marigold, or lavender to 1¼ cups or 300 ml of boiling water, and allow to brew for up to 10 minutes with the lid on the teapot. Cool.

Blend all into a smooth and delicious smoothie.

Very Berry-beetbucha

Blackcurrants contain large amounts of fiber, antioxidants, vitamins A, C, and K, and folic acid. In addition, the pips are also a source of gamma-linolenic acid, vitamin E, and important polyunsaturated fatty acids, whose benefits include being able to lower cholesterol levels. Maximum health benefits are derived from crushing the seeds or eating them in the form of blackcurrant powder.

MAKES 2 GLASSES

3½ oz / 100 g blackcurrants, frozen

1¾ cups / 50 g blueberries, frozen

1¾ cups / 50 g blackberries, frozen

1¾ cups / 50 g raspberries, frozen

1 tsp cinnamon, ground

1⅔ cups / 400 ml kefir or Greek yogurt

1 tbsp flax or hempseed oil, raw

1 red beet, pre-cooked

2 tbsp hemp seeds, shelled

1–2 Medjool dates, pitted

Blend all the ingredients into a smooth consistency.

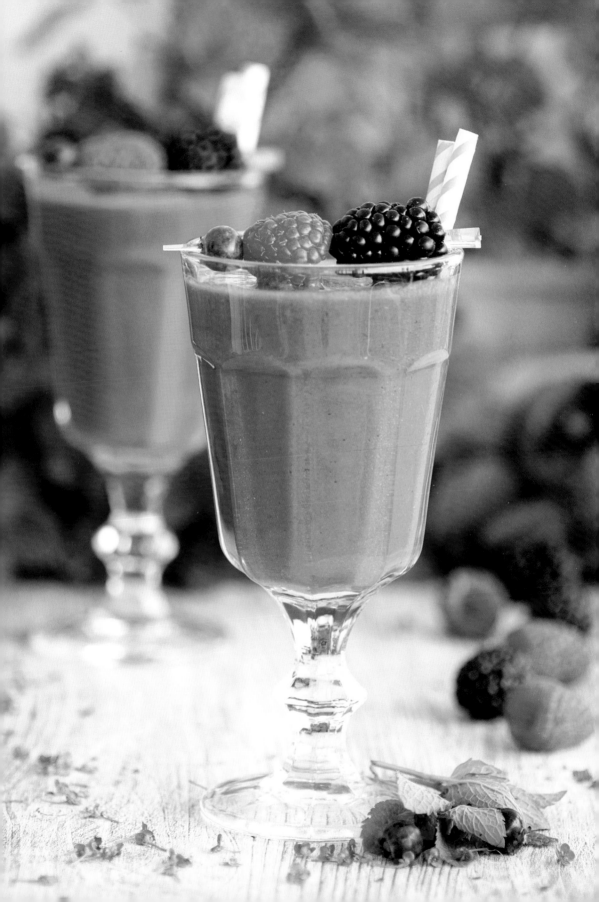

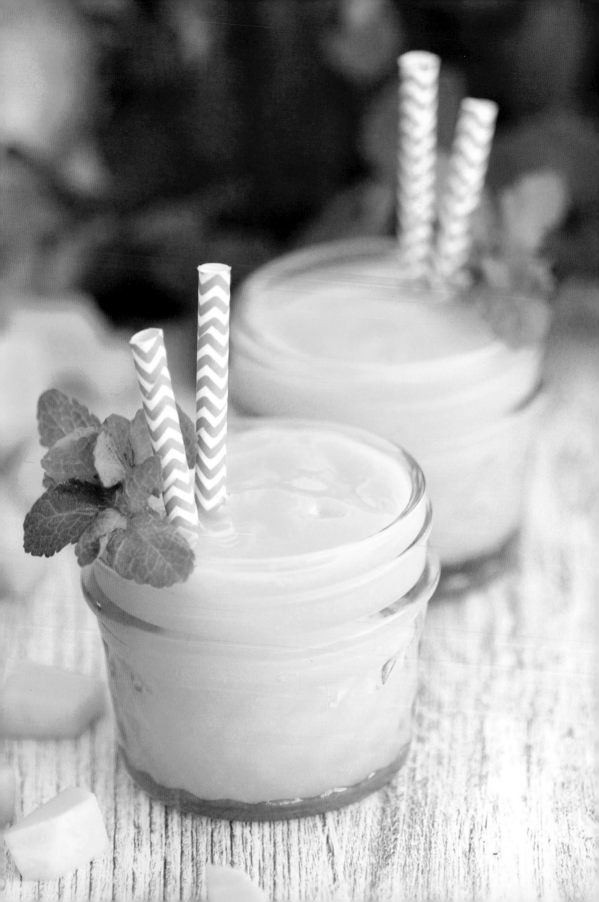

Gingered Mangorita

Mango is the national fruit of India and Pakistan, and is rich in several groups of antioxidants, such as beta-carotene, vitamin C, and potassium. It is particularly rich in beta-carotene, which is converted to vitamin A in the body. Vitamin A is good for eyesight, bones, skin, the mucous membranes, and the immune system. In addition to its positive effects on the body, beta-carotene is also very good for the skin. The antioxidant vitamin C also strengthens blood vessels, skin, teeth, and bones.

Like cashew nuts, mango contains urushiol, and those with allergies should be a little cautious, particularly when handling the skin.

TIP
If your blender is not very powerful, allow the mango to defrost a little before using.

MAKES 2 GLASSES

11 oz / 300 g mango, frozen

1–2 tsp ginger, grated

zest of ½ lime

1⅔ cups / 400 ml kombucha, plain

7 tbsp / 100 ml water

Blend all ingredients into a frosty and refreshing summer drink.

Stinging Nettle Elixir

Most people are familiar with stinging nettles. We have surely all had the experience of being stung at some time? And yet, few plants are as useful as stinging nettles.

In the 16th and 17th centuries, stinging nettles were used as medication for paralysis, rheumatism, scurvy, consumption, coughs, and baldness (as the leaves are hairy). Unfortunately, the desired results were not always achieved, even if the vitamins and minerals were doubtless much-needed additions to the diet. Nettles are now believed to have a purifying effect on the blood and to act as a general tonic for the body.

The highest level of nutrients is in the first leaves of the spring. Nettles are particularly rich in chlorophyll but also contain large amounts of beta-carotene, calcium, potassium, magnesium, iron, silica, manganese, flavonoids, provitamin A, vitamins C, K, and B, and folic acid. Powdered stinging nettles are easy to use and are available in health food stores. A teaspoonful of nettle powder is said to provide a whole day's vitamin C requirement.

MAKES 2 GLASSES

1 oz / 30 g spinach

1 pear, cored

½–1 tsp ginger, grated

2–3 tsp nettle powder (or a handful of fresh, soaked for an hour beforehand)

1 cup / 250 ml kombucha, plain

1 cup / 250 ml apple juice, freshly pressed

Blend all the ingredients into a wonderful green smoothie.

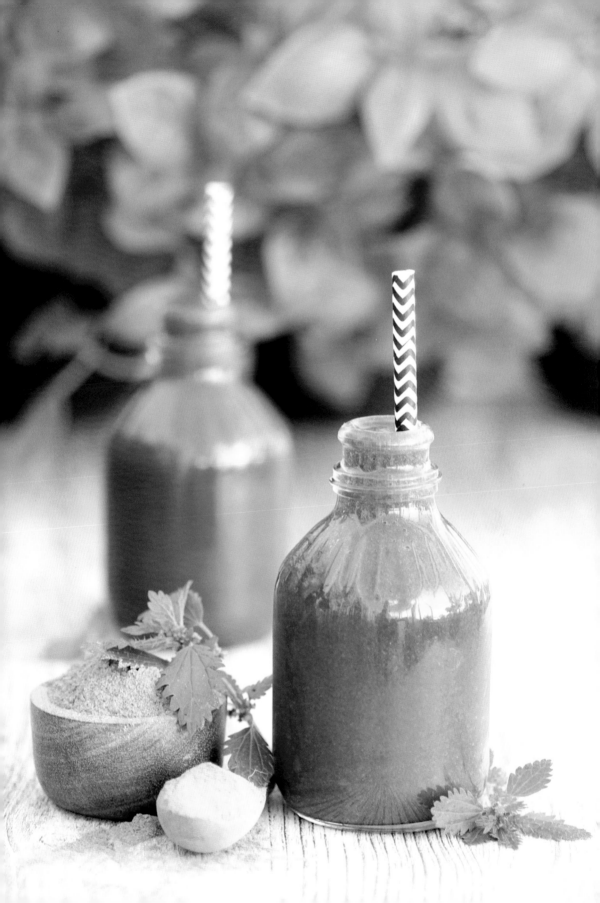

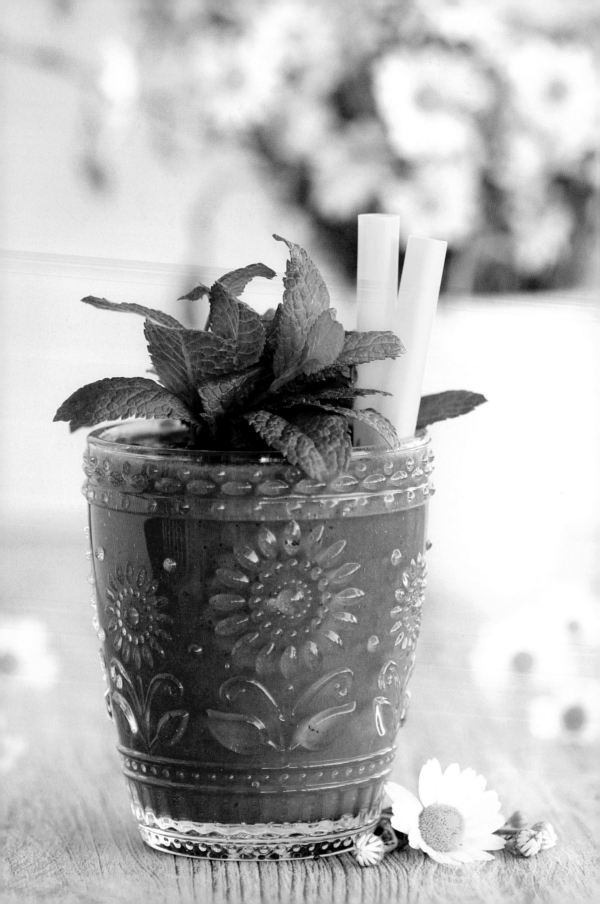

Mean Green Power Machine

Spirulina contains 60–70 percent protein, which is six times more than eggs and three times more than steak. The protein consists of 18 different amino acids, of which eight are essential to life. Spirulina also contains many important minerals, including calcium, magnesium, sodium, potassium, phosphorus, iodine, selenium, iron, copper, and zinc, a broad spectrum of B vitamins, such as vitamins B1, B2, B5, B6, B11, and B12, and vitamins C and E. Its beta-carotene content—beta-carotene is converted to vitamin A in the body—is 15 times higher than that of carrots and 40–60 times higher than that of spinach.

TIP
Increase to up to 2 teaspoonfuls of spirulina powder if you want an even healthier version. Be careful, though, as spirulina has a strong taste – it is best to start with small amounts so that your taste buds have a chance to get accustomed to it.

MAKES 2 GLASSES

2 oz / 60 g spinach

1–2 tsp ginger, grated

½ avocado

9 oz / 250 g pineapple, frozen

1⅔ cups / 400 ml kombucha

1 tsp spirulina powder

1 tsp wheatgrass powder

Blend all the ingredients into a wonderful green smoothie.

Burning Beet Magic Meal

I hope you are not throwing away the most nutritious part of the beet. Most of the nutritional value is in the tops, so do make use of them. If you have bought organic beets or have grown them yourself, this detox juice is a good way of using up the tops. Ask for extra tops if you are buying direct from the grower.

Beet tops are very similar to mangold in terms of both their taste and appearance.

MAKES 2 GLASSES

14 oz / 400 g red beets, pre-cooked

pinch of cayenne pepper

½ tsp Himalayan salt

tbsp olive oil, extra virgin

1–2 cloves garlic

1 cup / 250 ml kombucha, plain

Blend all the ingredients into a wonderful red smoothie.

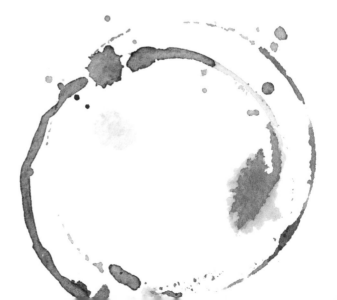

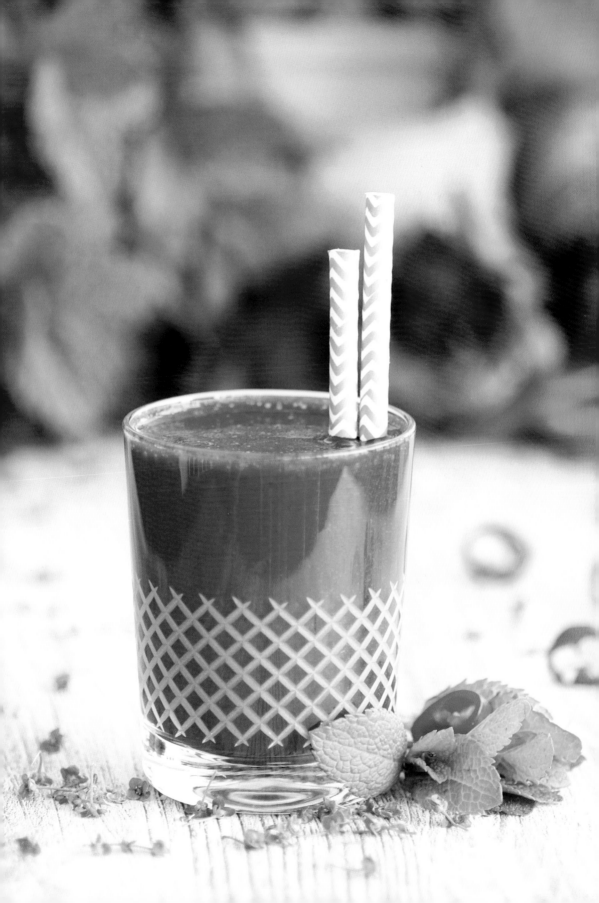

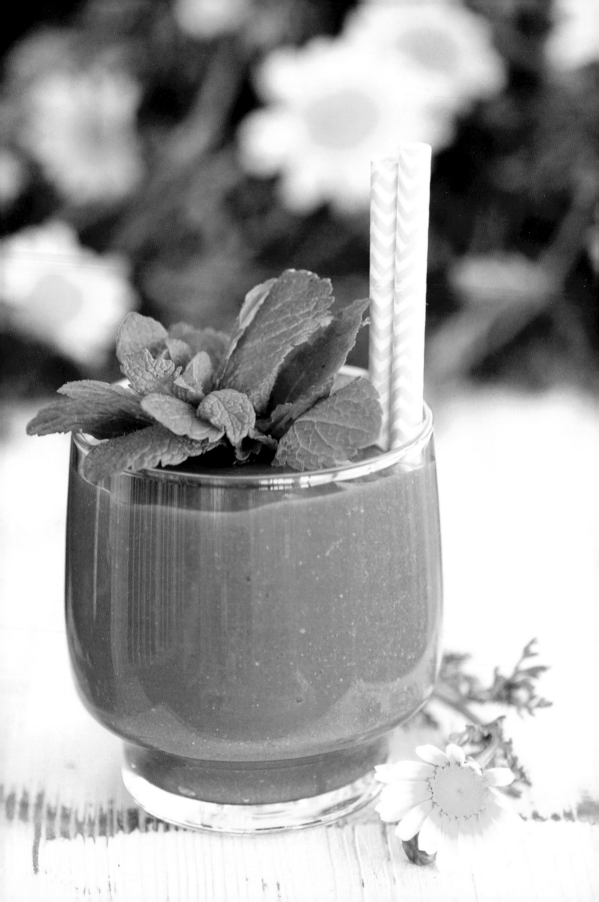

Carrot Coconut Power Meal

Carrots contain beta-carotene, a precursor to vitamin A. Vitamin A and carotene guard against cataracts and age-related changes to the retina, and are good for night vision. Lack of vitamin A can cause night blindness. Carrots are also good for the skin.

Carrots are best stored without their tops in a plastic bag in the fridge or in a cool room. Cut off the tops, otherwise they will use up nutrients and the carrots will go soft. Carrot tops are perfectly edible, just like beet tops—I often blend them into my smoothies in place of other greens.

TIP
This salad smoothie can be served as a soup, the perfect snack or a light lunch. Serve the soup in a bowl topped with fresh cilantro. Yum!

MAKES 2 GLASSES

4 large carrots, grated

handful fresh cilantro

3 tbsp olive oil, extra virgin

2 tsp ginger, grated

¼ chili

1 tsp curry powder

1–2 Medjool dates

Himalayan salt

1 cup / 250 ml coconut milk

⅔ cup / 150 ml kombucha, plain

Blend all the ingredients into a delicious smoothie.

Elixir of Life

Wheatgrass is rich in natural A and C vitamins, and particularly rich in B vitamins. It is also an excellent source of calcium, iron, magnesium, phosphorus, potassium, sodium, sulfur, cobalt, zinc, and proteins. Wheatgrass is also said to purify the blood and lower blood pressure—the juice reduces the amount of toxins in the body and supplies the blood with iron, improving circulation. Wheatgrass does not contain gluten.

Growing your own wheatgrass is simple. Soak the grain and allow it to sprout for one or two days, changing the water frequently. Spread out a ½–¾ inch layer of compost in a seed tray, pat it down and wet it thoroughly. Cover the compost with a layer of the sprouting grain, but do not push the grain down into the compost. Spray with water several times a day for the first three days, and afterwards water as you would a potted plant. Make sure you keep it moist. Keep the tray in a light place. The wheatgrass is ready to use when it is about 7 inches high—harvest by cutting a handful close to the grain.

MAKES 2 GLASSES

a handful of fresh wheatgrass, chopped (or 2 tsp powdered)

7 tbsp / 100 ml coconut milk, organic and additive-free

7 oz / 250 g pineapple, frozen

2–3 tsp ginger, grated

1 tsp coconut oil, extra virgin

1 cup / 250 ml kombucha

Blend all the ingredients into an elixir of life. I drink this almost every day, although when I make it, I double the amount of ginger and use three times as much wheatgrass.

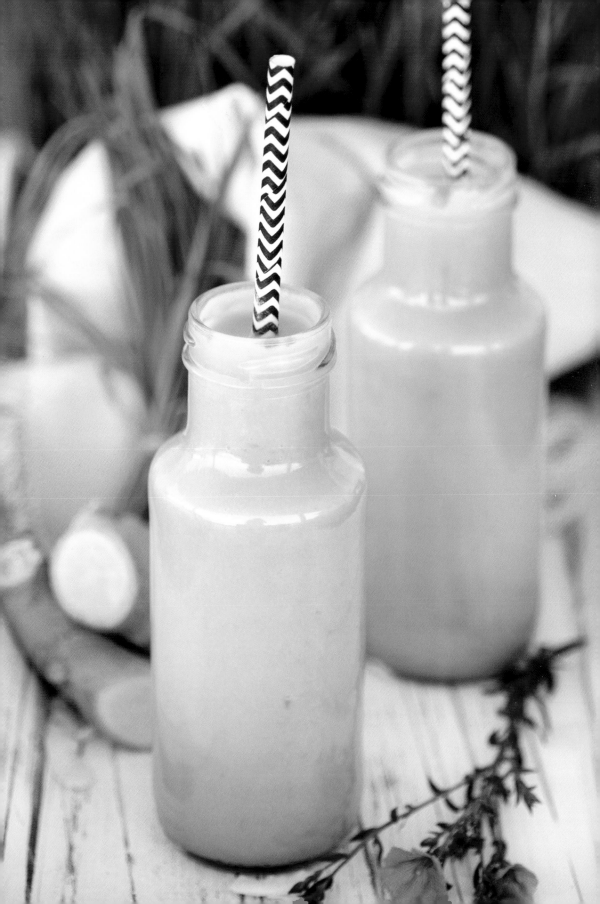

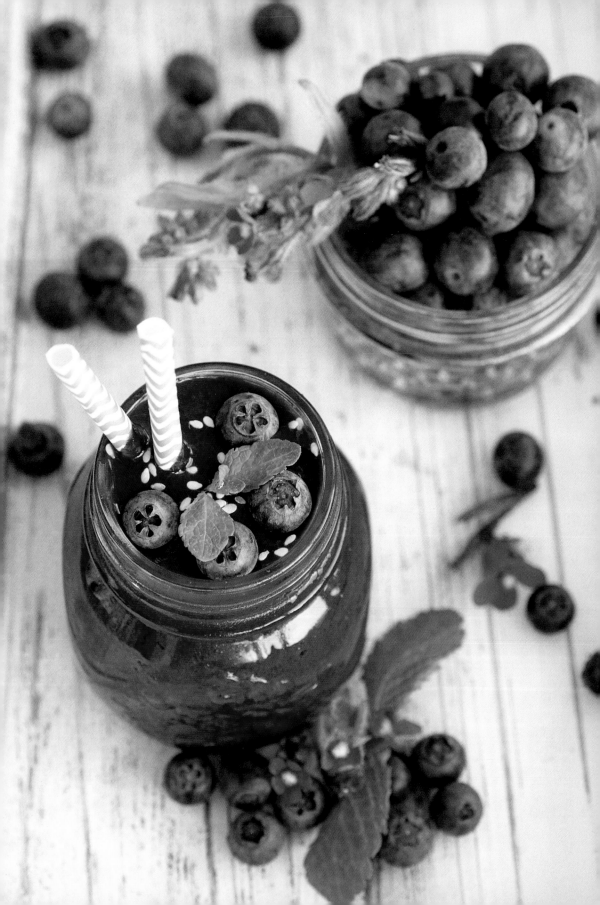

Minty Maple Blueberry Mojito

Maple syrup comes from the raw sap of the maple tree, which is sometimes also called maple water. The sap is collected at the beginning of spring and is then boiled down over a low heat until it turns into a golden-brown syrup. The sap, which is 2–3 per cent sugar, is tapped by drilling into the tree. The sugar comes from the tree's roots and rises up in the tree in the spring, giving the tree the energy to recover after the long winter. It is the evaporation process that makes maple water into maple syrup, and about 7½ gallons or 35 liters of maple water are needed to make one quart or one liter of syrup. Maple syrup is naturally rich in thiamine and in minerals such as zinc and calcium.

Unfortunately, there are several cheap brands of syrup, which, although flavored with maple essence, actually consist mainly of cheap corn syrup. These are not allowed to be labeled as maple syrup, but marketing departments can be ingenious so consumers should read the packaging before buying. If the label says pancake syrup, flavored syrup, maple essence, or something else and the cost is low, it is likely that it is not the real thing. The genuine article is 100 per cent maple syrup, and should ideally also be organic.

MAKES 2 GLASSES

1⅔ cups / 400 ml kombucha, plain

2 tsp chia seeds

9 oz / 250 g blueberries, wild and frozen

2–3 tsp mint, chopped

2–3 tbsp maple syrup

Soak the chia seeds in the kombucha for 10–15 minutes. Add the other ingredients and blend to make a delicious, dark purple, probiotic smoothie.

Raspberry Peach Dream

Peaches belong to the same family as plums, almonds, and apricots. There are several thousand different varieties; most of them have downy skin but there are also smooth-skinned varieties called nectarines.

Peaches are mainly imported from Italy, but also come from Greece and Spain, with the main season being July to September.

Unripe fruit should be stored at room temperature, while ripe peaches should be kept in a cold place at 35–39 °F / 2–4 °C for as little time as possible as they have a short shelf life. Peaches are delicate and very easily damaged.

I usually buy large quantities when they are in season, leave them until they are perfectly ripe, then pit and quarter them, and store them in the freezer—great in the winter for smoothies or jam or for baking.

MAKES 2 GLASSES

3 peaches, pitted

9 oz / 250 g raspberries, frozen

1–2 Medjool dates, pitted

1⅔ cups / 400 ml kombucha, plain

Blend all the ingredients into a yummy smoothie.

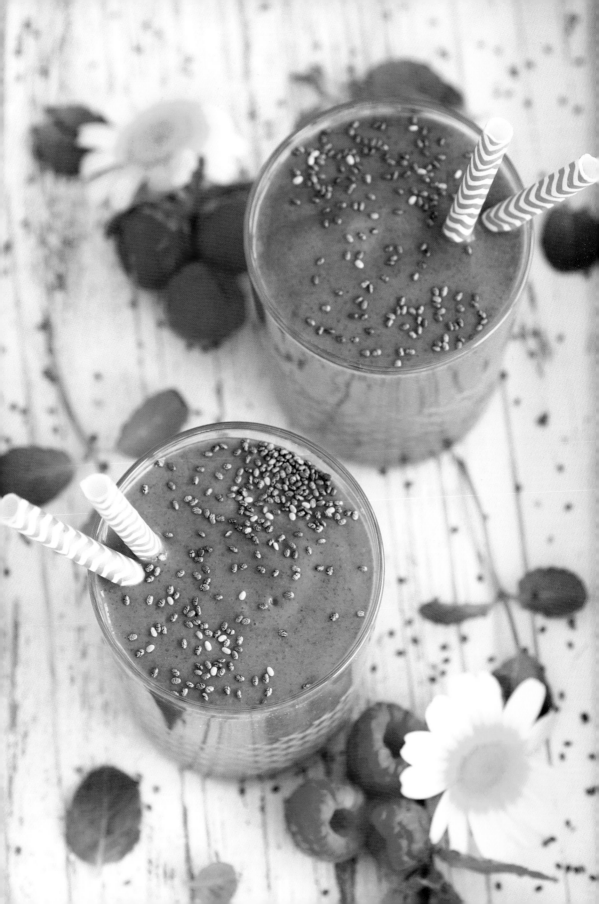

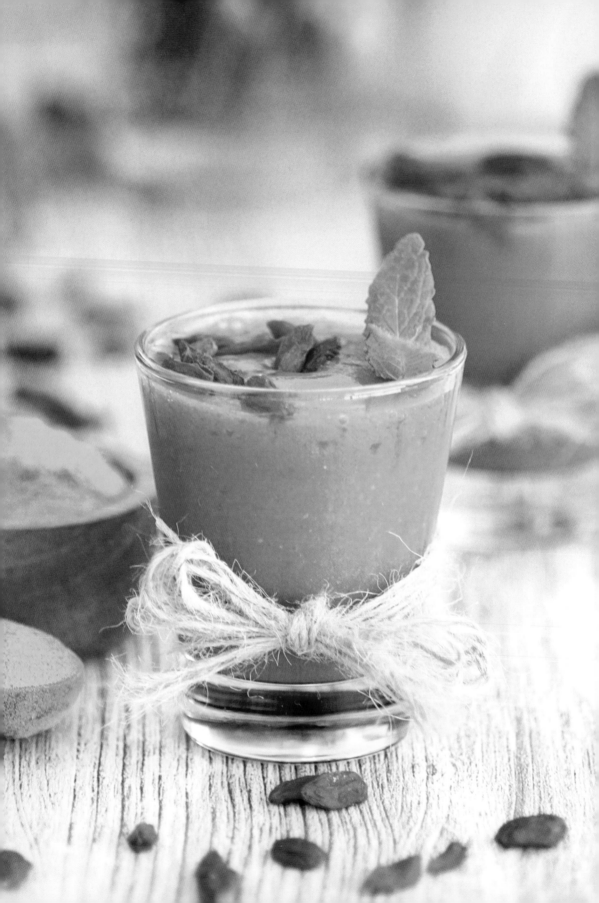

Buddha's Delight

In the past, green tea was used as a medication; nowadays, it is drunk mainly because it is delicious and healthy. Green tea is common in China and Japan, but it is now drunk throughout the world.

It is actually made from the same tealeaves as are used for black tea, but with green tea the leaves are not allowed to oxidize. This gives the tea more of a vegetable taste suggestive of hay, grass, algae, or the sea. For this reason, green tea can take a bit of getting used to in comparison with the more readily available black tea.

Green tea contains a lot of polyphenols, antioxidants that are said to protect the body's cells and DNA against the free radicals that can cause cell damage, cell death, aging, and age-related diseases.

The tealeaves retain much of the goodness found naturally in the leaves, including large amounts of useful antioxidants, vitamins, and minerals. The tea has a low theine content and is well suited to use in detoxes. Buy organic if you can.

MAKES 2 GLASSES

1 cup / 250 ml green tea, cooled

4 tbsp goji berries

1–2 tsp ginger, grated

1 cup / 250 ml kombucha, plain

ice

Make the tea according to the instructions and cool. Soak the goji berries in the cold tea for 10–15 minutes; I usually soak them direct in the blender. Blend all the ingredients into a spicy smoothie. For a cold smoothie, add in some ice at the end.

113

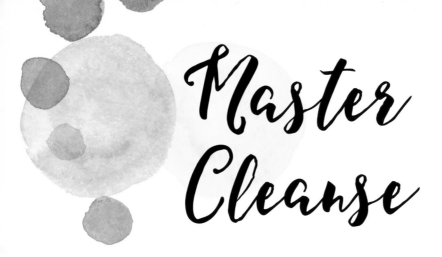

Master Cleanse

Chilis are a boost for the metabolism. Hotness varies from chili to chili, so you need to be a little careful. The most common varieties in Europe are cayenne peppers, aji chili peppers, bonnet peppers, perennial cayenne peppers, and rocoto chili peppers. Dried chili is also available in jars or packets and is almost as good as fresh chili. But be careful with the heat.

The heat in chilis is not in the seeds but in the membrane that holds the seeds. So you can reduce the hotness by halving the chili lengthwise and scraping out the insides with a knife. The substance that makes chilis hot is called capsaicin. It is a water-insoluble oil, so if your mouth gets too hot, drinking water will not help. On the other hand, capsaicin is fat soluble, so eating something like nuts will bring relief.

MAKES 2 GLASSES

2 apples, cored

2 tbsp maple syrup

zest of 1 lime

pinch or two cayenne pepper

1⅔ cups / 400 ml kombucha, plain

ice

Blend all the ingredients into a spicy smoothie. For a cold smoothie, add ice at the end.

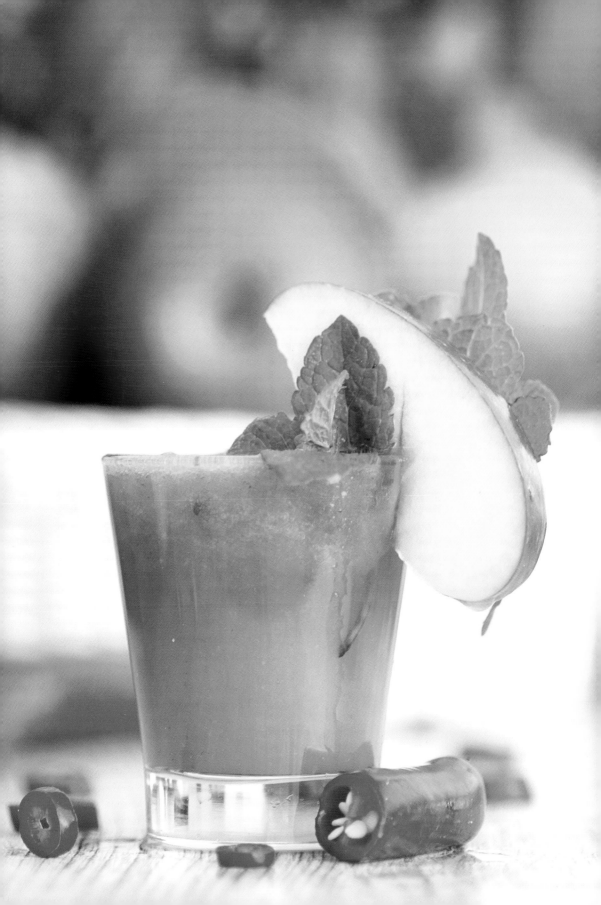

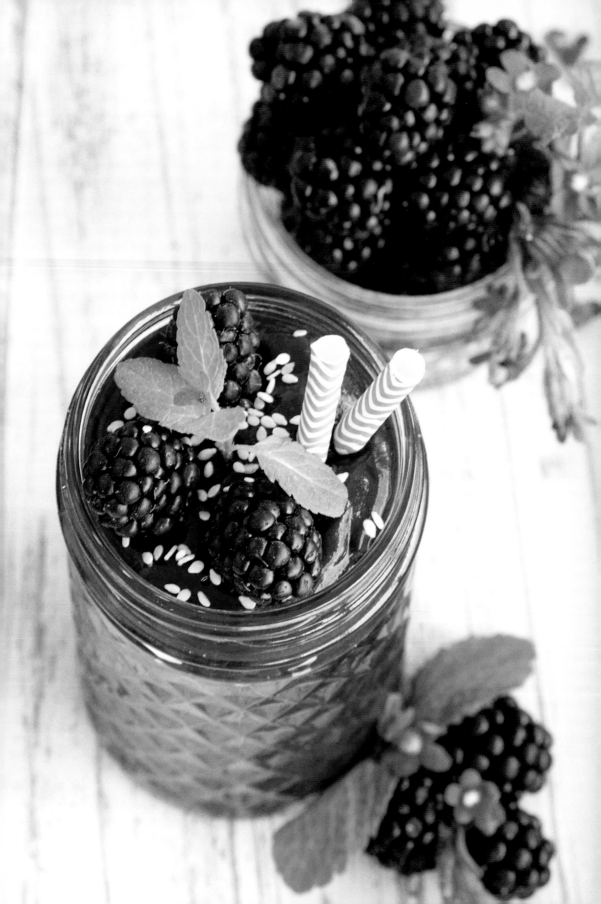

Black Magic

The chaga mushroom (*Inonotus obliquus*) is known in Siberia as "The Mushroom of Immortality," "A Gift from God," or "A Gift from Heaven." Chaga has been used in Asia for several thousand years to strengthen the immune system.

Scientific studies have shown that chaga may have a beneficial effect on breast cancer, liver cancer, uterine cancer, and stomach cancer as well as on high blood pressure and diabetes. Chaga has also been shown to be helpful for almost all cases of psoriasis. Chaga is good for type 2 diabetes because it lowers blood sugar levels, which means that less insulin is needed.

It is said to be antibacterial, antifungal, anti-candida, and antiviral. It also keeps the immune system in balance and so is good for autoimmune diseases. You cannot over-dose on chaga.

I make tea, decoctions, and extract, and use chaga powder in my smoothies.

MAKES 2 GLASSES

1 cup / 250 ml chaga tea, cooled

1¾ oz / 50 g cashew nuts, natural

2 tsp hemp seeds, shelled

11 oz / 300 g blackberries, frozen

½ tsp cinnamon, ground

1–2 Medjool dates, pitted

1 cup / 250 ml kefir of your choice

Make the tea according to the instructions and cool. Blend the cashews with the tea first, then add the other ingredients, and blend into a magical smoothie.

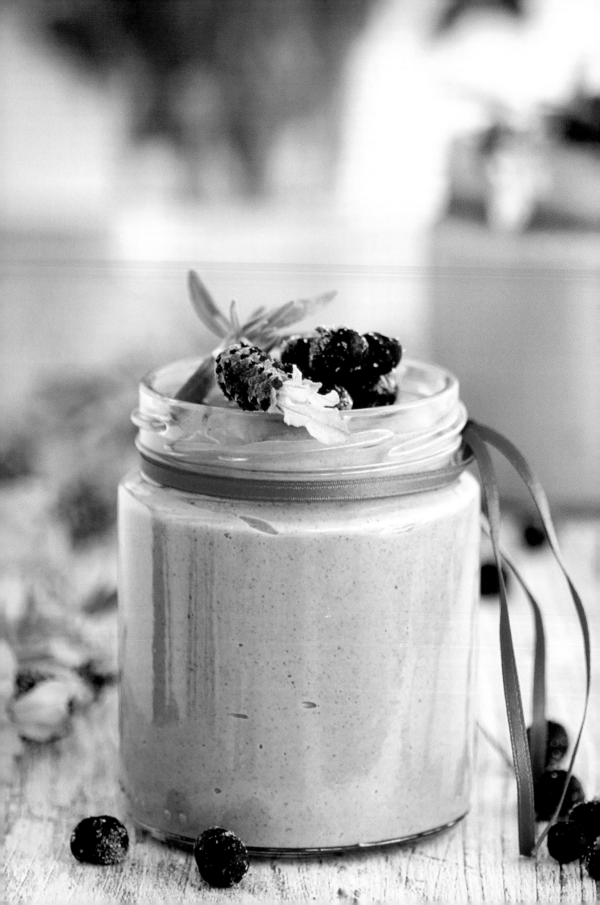

Blueberry Lavender Bliss

Lavender is said to be an antispasmodic and a diuretic, and is believed to relieve diarrhea and irritation of the stomach and intestines. It can also be used to heal wounds, and as it irritates the skin and increases blood flow, it can also relieve lower back pain, other muscle pain, and rheumatic disorders. The essential oil is also antiseptic, calming, and can soothe insect bites and minor burns. To soothe a headache, apply a drop of oil to the temples. Six drops of oil in the bathwater will calm anxious children so they go to sleep more easily.

A mixture of dried lavender flowers can be used to calm worries, dizziness, and migraine. You can, for example, make your own lavender tea by pouring a generous ¾ cup or 200 ml of hot water onto 2 teaspoonfuls of lavender flowers and allowing it to brew for five minutes. Cold lavender tea will keep in the fridge in a sealed glass bottle for up to a week.

MAKES 2 GLASSES

1 cup / 250 ml lavender tea, cooled

2 tbsp chia seeds

1 cup / 250 ml natural Greek yogurt with live culture

7 oz / 200 g blueberries, wild

1–2 Medjool dates, pitted

Make the tea and cool. Soak the chia seeds in the cold lavender tea for 10–15 minutes. Blend all the ingredients into a delicious smoothie.

Nordic Love Story

Lingonberries are one of the commonest wild berries in the Nordic region, and the plants can withstand temperatures as low as –40 degrees, even though the foliage is evergreen. Although most lingonberries grow in the wild, you can also grow them in your garden if you have the right conditions.

Lingonberries contain large amounts of vitamins A, B, and C, and the minerals potassium, calcium, phosphorus, and iron. They are bactericidal and are therefore, like cranberries, effective against urinary tract infections. The berries also neutralize the smell of urine. Lingonberries can also help gastric ulcers and inflamed gums. They used to be sold at drugstores, for uses such as reducing fever.

MAKES 2 GLASSES

1⅔ cups / 400 ml kefir or yogurt, Greek-style

7 oz / 200 g lingonberries, frozen

1 tsp cinnamon

½ tsp cardamom

2–3 tbsp raw honey

1 tsp bee pollen

Blend all the ingredients into a dreamy pink smoothie.

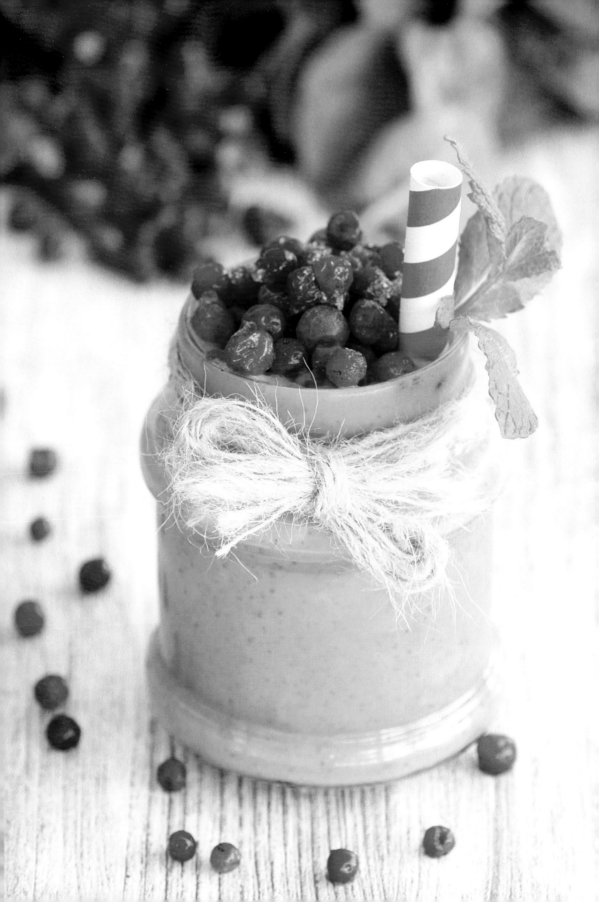

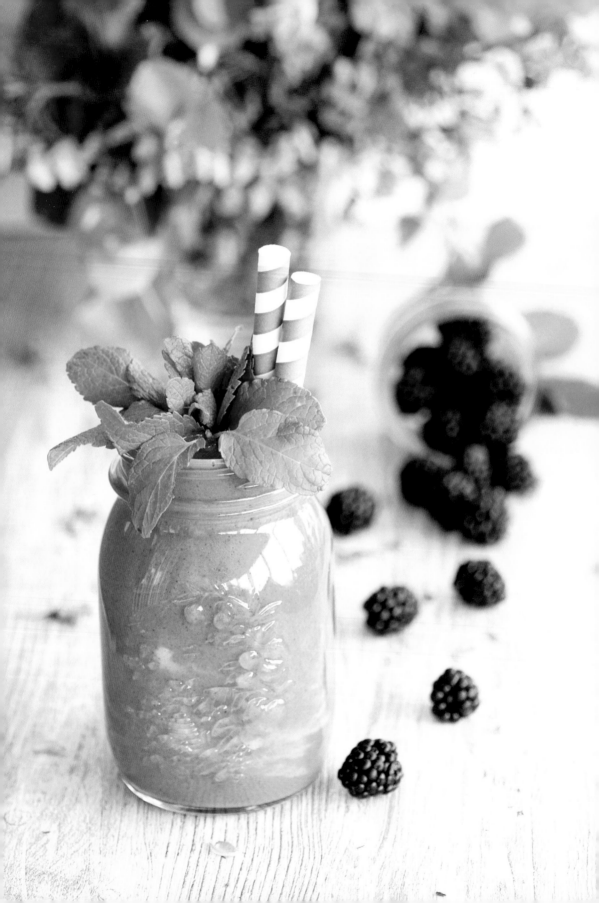

Blackberry Beast

A handful of blackberries contains almost half the recommended daily intake of fiber. Fiber keeps the bowels active and promotes digestion. They also help to regulate blood sugar. Blackberries are also a good source of vitamins C and E, potassium, manganese, magnesium, iron, and vitamin K, which helps the body take up calcium.

The blackberry's dark color comes from anthocyanins, chemical pigments and antioxidants that can reduce inflammation in the body and protect it against free radicals that may otherwise damage cells and contribute to causing cancer.

MAKES 2 GLASSES

2 tsp flaxseeds

⅔ cup / 150 ml apple juice, freshly pressed

1 cup / 250 ml kefir or yogurt, Greek-style

9 oz / 250 g blackberries, frozen

1 tsp chaga powder (optional)

½ tsp vanilla powder or extract

Soak the flaxseeds in the apple juice for 10–15 minutes. Blend all the ingredients into a fluffy smoothie.

Melonberry

Melon belongs to the same family as pumpkin and cucumber. There are many different varieties of melon, and they are normally divided into watermelons and muskmelons. Watermelons usually have red flesh and brownish-black seeds. There are also seedless varieties and types with yellow or orange flesh. In contrast to watermelons, muskmelon seeds sit in the middle of the fruit, which makes them easier to remove. Muskmelons generally have smoother flesh and a sweeter, more scented, flavor. Common varieties of muskmelon include honeydew, cantaloupe, charentais, and galia melons.

MAKES 2 GLASSES

2 tsp chia seeds

⅔ cup / 150 ml kombucha

11 oz / 300 g watermelon, cubed

⅔ cup / 150 g raspberries, frozen

3½ oz / 100 g strawberries, frozen

1 banana

1 tsp lúcuma powder (optional)

Soak the chia seeds in the kombucha for 10–15 minutes. Blend everything into a smooth consistency.

TIP
If your blender is less powerful, allow the berries to defrost a little beforehand.

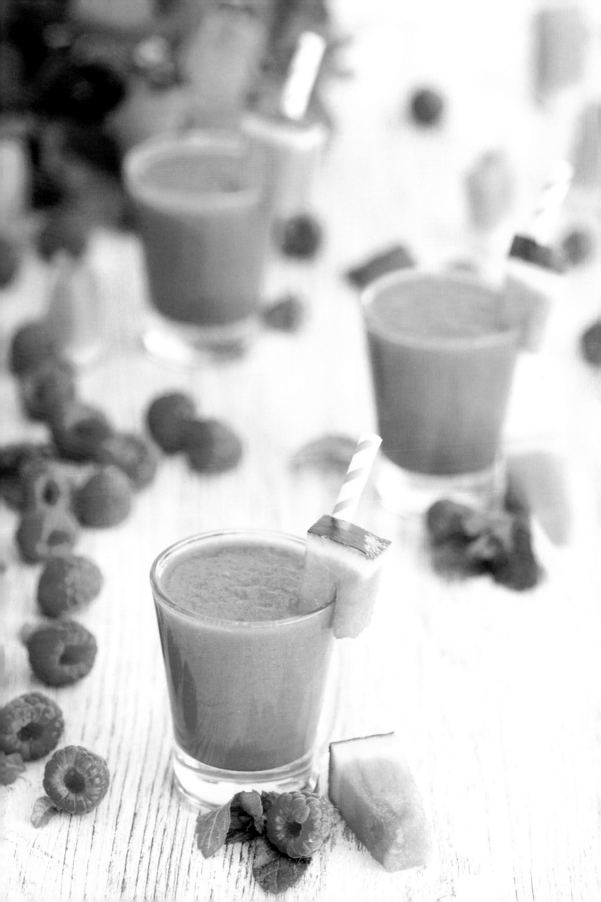

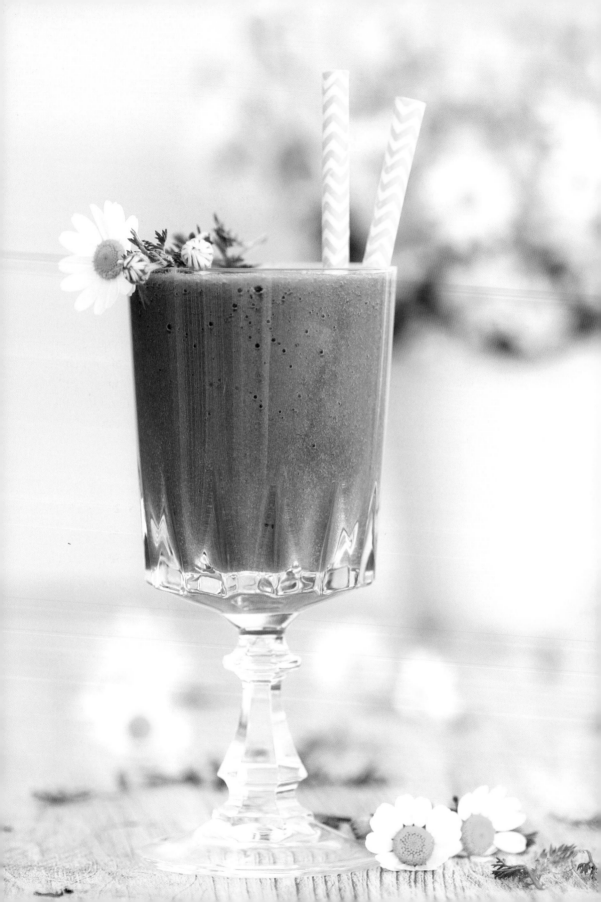

Green First Aid

Fresh parsley leaves contain minerals such as iron, calcium, potassium, and magnesium, and also vitamins A and C. Five grams of parsley provides our daily requirement of vitamin A and one ounce or 30 grams provides our daily requirement of vitamin C. Parsley is a diuretic and an antispasmodic, lowers blood pressure, and can possibly reduce the risk of irregular heart activity (atrial fibrillation). It also stimulates the appetite and boosts the metabolism. Chewing parsley makes the breath fresher—useful for countering the smell of garlic.

MAKES 2 GLASSES

1 oz / 30 g parsley leaves, chopped

1 oz / 30 g spinach

1–2 tsp ginger, grated

2 kiwifruit, peeled and chopped

3 pears, cored

1 cup / 250 ml kombucha or water kefir

ice as needed

Blend all ingredients into a delicious green drink. For a cold smoothie, blend in a few ice cubes at the end.

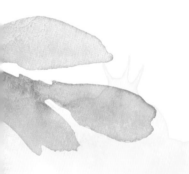

Passionate Raspberry Romance

Raspberries contain all sorts of beneficial ingredients that keep us fit and healthy. These superberries are anti-inflammatory, strengthen the immune system, and are said to guard against cancer and heart disease. Raspberries are rich in fiber, which helps in keeping cholesterol levels down. They contain large amounts of vitamin C, folic acid, iron, calcium, and potassium. Raspberries also have an expectorant and detoxifying effect, and can help relieve menstrual pain.

Buy raspberries that have an even color. They can be easily damaged and should be used within two days. Stock up when they are in season and store in the freezer. You can also buy freeze-dried raspberry powder in health food stores which works well in smoothies.

TIP
If you have a less powerful blender, allow the raspberries to defrost a little before using.

MAKES 2 GLASSES

4 passion fruit

9 oz / 250 g raspberries, frozen

1 banana

2–3 tsp coconut nectar sugar (or raw honey)

1⅔ cups / 400 ml kombucha, plain

Scoop out the passion fruit flesh, add to the other ingredients, and blend everything into a tasty smoothie.

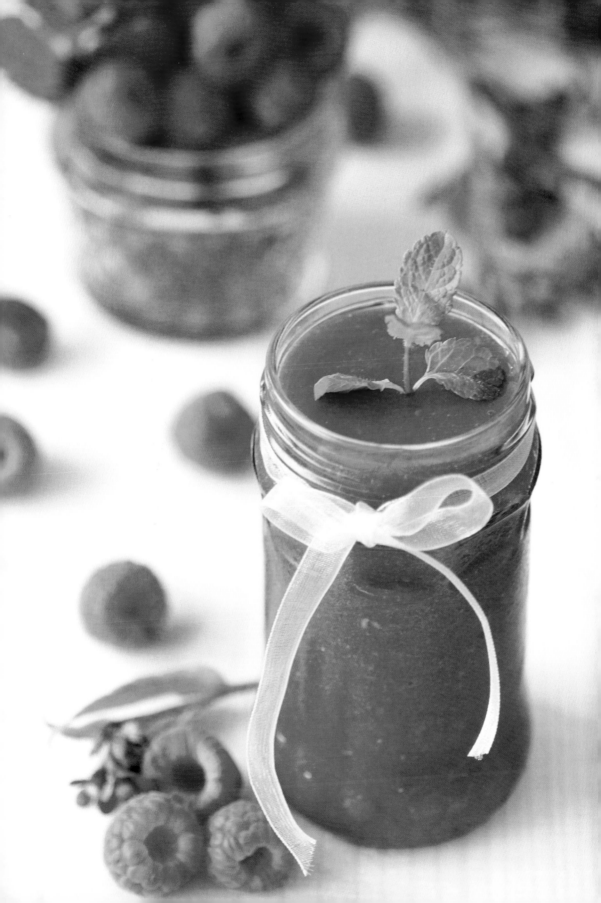

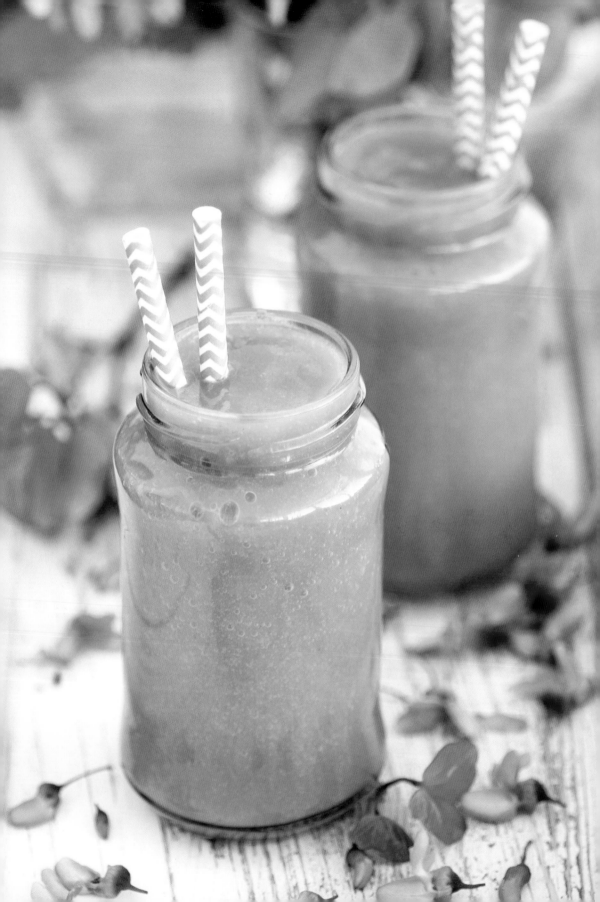

Mystical Garden

If you wash your kiwifruit, the skin is perfectly edible. It is soft and flavorsome, and you will not feel any hairiness in your mouth. It is also good for you. Kiwifruit contains large amounts of vitamins C and E. They do not combine well with dairy products, and should instead be blended with other berries and tropical fruit.

Until the 1960s, the kiwifruit was known as the Chinese gooseberry. Kiwis are commonly transported in from New Zealand, but we can also get them from the Mediterranean countries between November and April. A good kiwi should give a little when you press it. Watch out for kiwis that are too soft and may have an unpleasant taste.

MAKES 2 GLASSES

1 cup / 250 ml dandelion tea, cooled

1 cup / 250 ml water kefir

½–1 tsp ginger, freshly grated

3 kiwifruit, chopped

1 oz / 30 g spinach

Blend everything into a sweet and delicious, green smoothie.

Minty Mango Lassi

I just love mango lassi, a traditional South Asian drink, originally from the Punjab in India/Pakistan. It is made by combining yogurt, water, fruit, and spices such as ginger, cinnamon, nutmeg, chili, cumin, and cilantro into a frothy drink. You can make it with any fruit or berries you like.

Mint comes in several varieties and is recognized by its characteristic, fresh aroma and taste. The most common sort is peppermint, which is thought to be disinfectant, anti-spasmodic, anti-inflammatory, cooling, and calming, as well as good for the digestion. Spearmint has similar properties. Mint is very easy to grow, spreads readily, and can be very easily frozen or dried.

MAKES 2 GLASSES

1⅔ cups / 400 ml kefir or yogurt, natural

7 oz / 200 g mango, frozen

3–4 tsp mint, chopped

½ tsp cinnamon

½ tsp cardamom

pinch nutmeg

½ tsp ginger, ground

Blend everything into a delicious green drink and enjoy.

TIP
If your blender is less powerful, allow the mango to defrost a little beforehand.

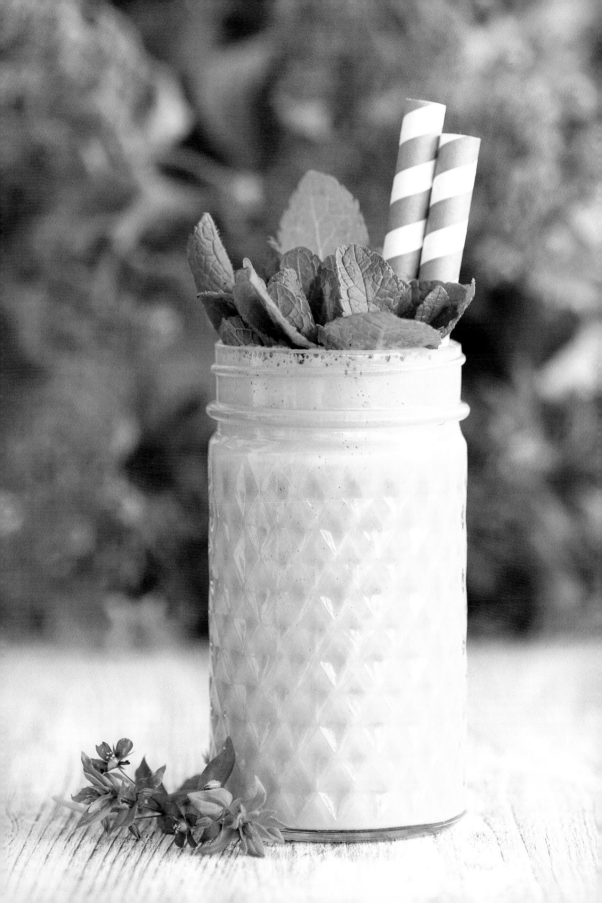

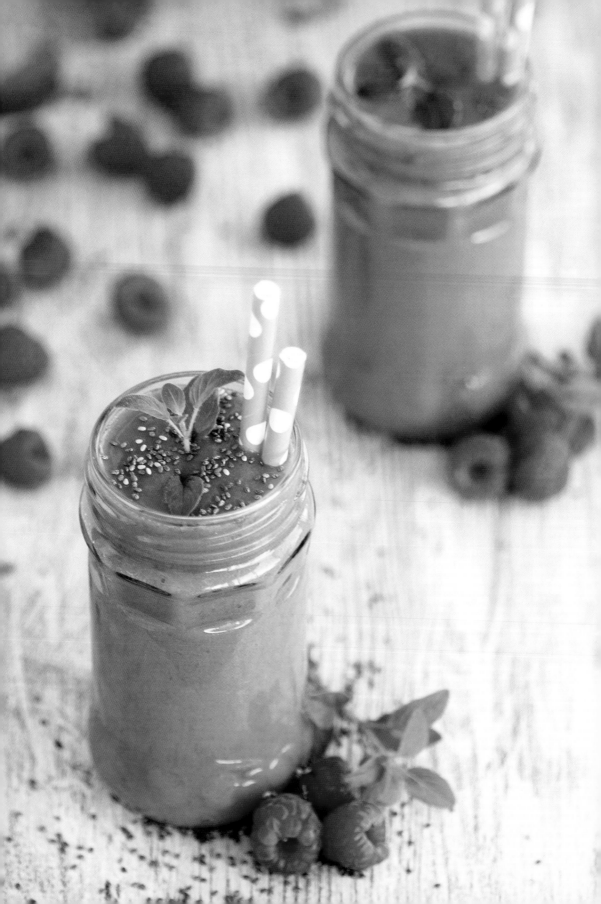

Hibiscus Heaven

It is said that hibiscus tea was drunk by the Pharaohs of ancient Egypt. It is a slightly tart, red-colored tea made from dried hibiscus flowers. It can be drunk either hot or cold and has a flavor sometimes likened to cranberry.

The tea is said to be calming and to have a slightly diuretic and antipyretic effect; it is also said to increase bile production and protect the mucous membranes. It lowers the blood pressure and stimulates bowel movements. It is rich in vitamin C and an antioxidant, and strengthens the immune system.

As hibiscus tea lowers blood pressure, it should not be drunk by those with low blood pressure. It should be completely avoided by anyone who is pregnant, as it is said to contain a certain amount of endocrine disrupters.

TIP
If your blender is not very powerful, allow the raspberries and mango to defrost before use.

MAKES 2 GLASSES

generous ¾ cup / 200 ml hibiscus tea, cooled

generous ¾ cup / 200 ml water kefir or kombucha

7 oz / 200 g raspberries, frozen

3½ oz / 100 g mango, frozen

1–2 tsp raw honey

Make the tea and allow to cool. Blend everything into a smooth consistency.

Love Potion

Pomegranate is a superfruit that comes originally from Persia and has been cultivated for thousands of years. It is particularly rich in folic acid and antioxidants such as vitamin C, carotene, gallocatechin, and anthocyanin (which gives pomegranates their pink color). The antioxidants build up the cells of the body and help to prevent disease. The folic acid is important for the growth of new cells and helps the body produce red blood cells.

Short of time, or having trouble extracting the tasty pomegranate seeds? Try juicing the pomegranates instead—the juice freezes well in ice-cube trays. Fresh pomegranates are available during the winter months, but you can also use frozen or dried pomegranate seeds out of season.

MAKES 2 GLASSES

1 cup / 250 ml pomegranate juice, freshly pressed

1 cup / 250 ml kombucha

7 oz / 200 g raspberries, frozen

⅔ cup / 150 g mango, frozen

Blend everything into a red love potion.

TIP
If your blender is less powerful, allow the raspberries and mango to defrost a little before use.

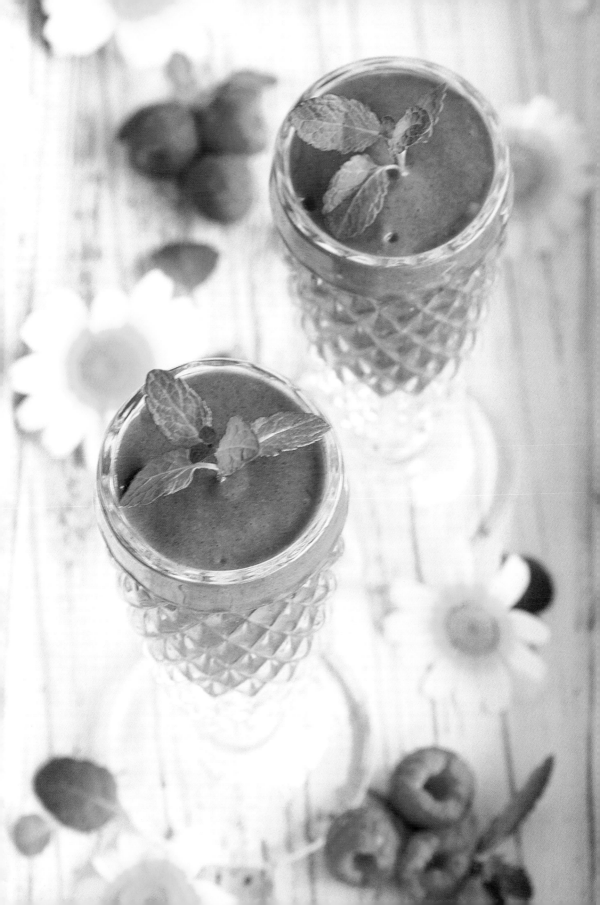

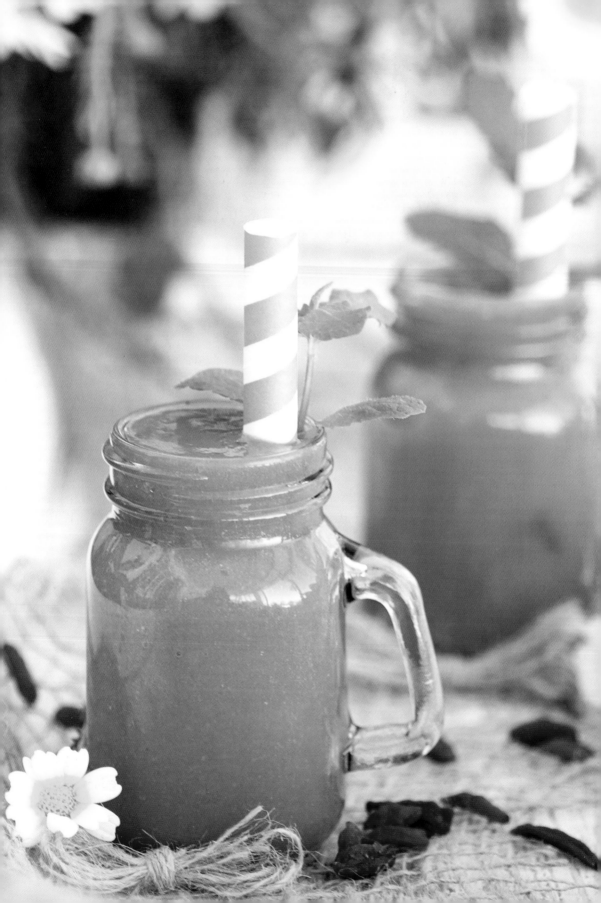

Morning Jump Start

Chia seeds are a true superfood. A 3½ ounce or 100-gram portion contains one ounce or 31 grams of fat, and as much as ¾ ounce or 20 grams of this is alpha-linolenic acid (ALA), the vegetable form of Omega-3 fatty acid. Two teaspoons of chia seeds contain more Omega-3 than a standard-size salmon fillet. Omega-3 is important for the body's hormonal balance and can have an anti-inflammatory effect. The seeds are also rich in minerals such as magnesium, potassium, and zinc.

A portion of 3½ ounces or 100 grams of chia seeds also contains ¾ ounce or 21 grams of protein, including no fewer than 18 amino acids. In other words, it is an important source of vegetable protein.

Chia seeds also contain large amounts of water-soluble fiber, which is beneficial to gut function and helps to stabilize blood sugar levels.

MAKES 2 GLASSES

2 tbsp chia seeds

4 tbsp goji berries

⅔ cup / 150 ml apple juice, freshly pressed

⅔ cup / 150 g strawberries, frozen

1 cup / 250 ml kefir

1 banana, frozen

Soak the chia seeds and goji berries in the apple juice for 10–15 minutes. Blend everything into a delicious vitamin C boost.

Total Detoxification

I have a large stock of spinach at home in my enormous freezer. I grow much of my spinach myself, and when there is more of the fresh variety than I can eat, I freeze it for use in the winter. I find it best to blend it first and then freeze it in ice-cube trays. I store the cubes in re-sealable bags, making a note of the contents and date. They will keep for up to six months.

Spinach is a superfood and a great source of antioxidants. The leaves are incredibly nutritious, and contain, amongst other things, vitamins A, C, E, K, and B9 (folic acid). Spinach is also rich in copper, iron, magnesium, calcium, chlorophyll, fiber, and other beneficial substances.

Spinach has a high inorganic nitrate content that is thought to improve physical performance and muscle development. Studies have shown that spinach makes the mitochondria—the energy hubs of the muscle cells—more efficient, thereby reducing the body's need for oxygen during physical exertion. Spinach is also believed to combat cancer and high blood pressure, and to be good for gastric ulcers.

MAKES 2 GLASSES

2 oz / 60 g spinach

1 oz / 30 g kale, stalks removed

1⅔ cups / 400 ml kombucha or water kefir

2 tsp wheatgrass powder

1 tsp spirulina powder

1–2 tsp ginger, grated

9 oz / 250 g pineapple, frozen

Blend the spinach and kale with the kombucha for a few moments, add the other ingredients, and blend until you have a delicious, green health drink.

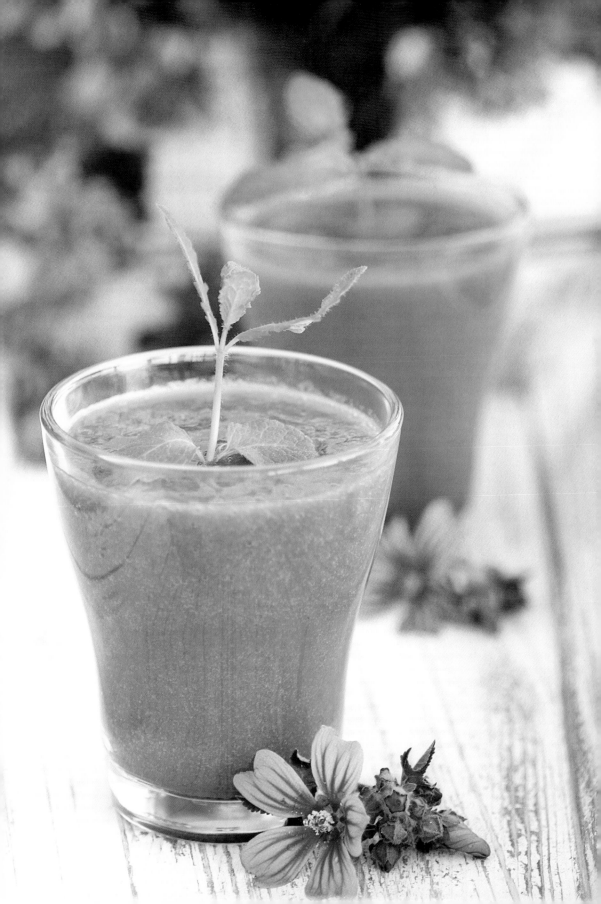

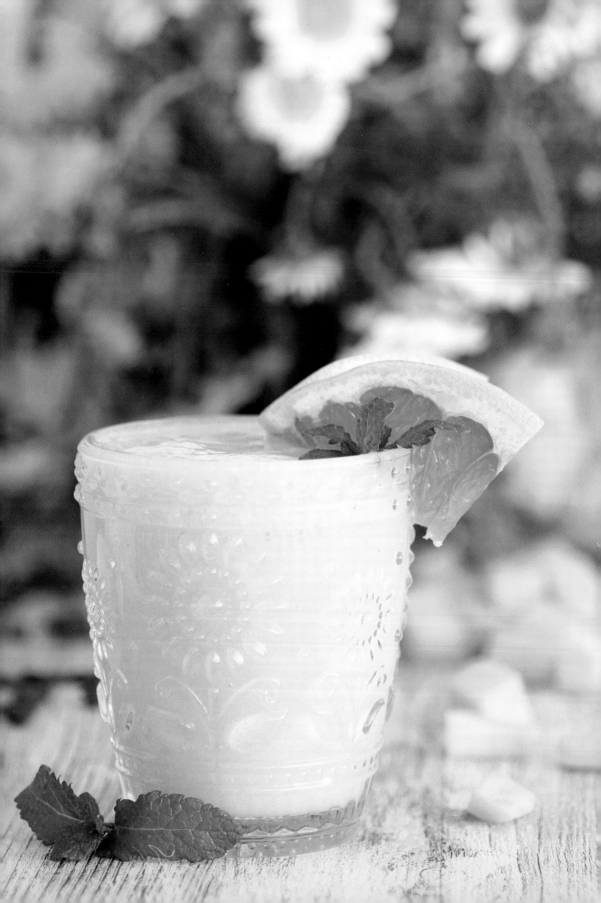

Rise and Shine

A grapefruit contains more than an adult's daily requirement of vitamin C. Pink and red grapefruits have a sweeter taste than yellow ones. Grapefruit gives the immune system a real boost, makes the skin glow, and contains lots of invigorating antioxidants that protect against cardiovascular disease and cancer. Grapefruit is good for flu, irritation of the mouth or throat, ear infections, and urinary tract infections. It helps to lower the "bad" LDL cholesterol and keep blood pressure down. Crushed grapefruit seeds have antifungal and antibacterial properties, and can be used to treat fungal infections.

Grapefruit may affect the working of certain drugs, particularly those for heart and blood pressure disorders, so if you are taking medication you should check with your doctor before you start regularly eating grapefruit.

MAKES 2 GLASSES

2 tsp chia seeds

1 cup / 250 ml kombucha, plain

4 grapefruit

⅔ cup / 150 g pineapple, frozen

1 tbsp maca powder

1 tbsp lúcuma powder

Soak the chia seeds in the kombucha for 10–15 minutes. Peel and segment the grapefruit, making sure that none of the membrane, pips, or peel go into the smoothie. Blend everything into a delicious smoothie.

Witches Brew

In the past, rose hips were used in folk medicine to prevent scurvy, or vitamin C deficiency. Rose hips have also been considered effective against constipation, fatigue, joint problems, diverticulosis, emphysema, ear problems, hemorrhoids, bladder problems, colic, stiffness, and problems with the back, legs, feet, and neck. Rose hips have not just been used to treat humans; they have also been given to horses to enhance their immune systems.

Whole rose hip powder is made from whole, dried rose hips and contains 60 times as much vitamin C as citrus fruit. It is also rich in antioxidants and vital minerals such as iron, calcium, potassium, and magnesium. Rose hip also contains a large amount of folic acid, which is particularly helpful for breastfeeding women or those trying for a baby. Making your own rose hip powder is simple: dry whole rose hips and grind them to a powder.

MAKES 2 GLASSES

1 cup / 250 ml dandelion tea, cooled

2 apples, cored

2 tbsp pumpkin puree

3 tsp whole rose hip powder

2 tsp chaga powder

1 tsp maca powder

1 tsp lúcuma powder

1 cup / 250 ml kombucha or water kefir

Make the tea and cool. Blend all the ingredients into a magical health drink.

NOTE
Fresh stinging nettles work well in this smoothie too, but soak the crisp leaves in water for 30 minutes to an hour beforehand.

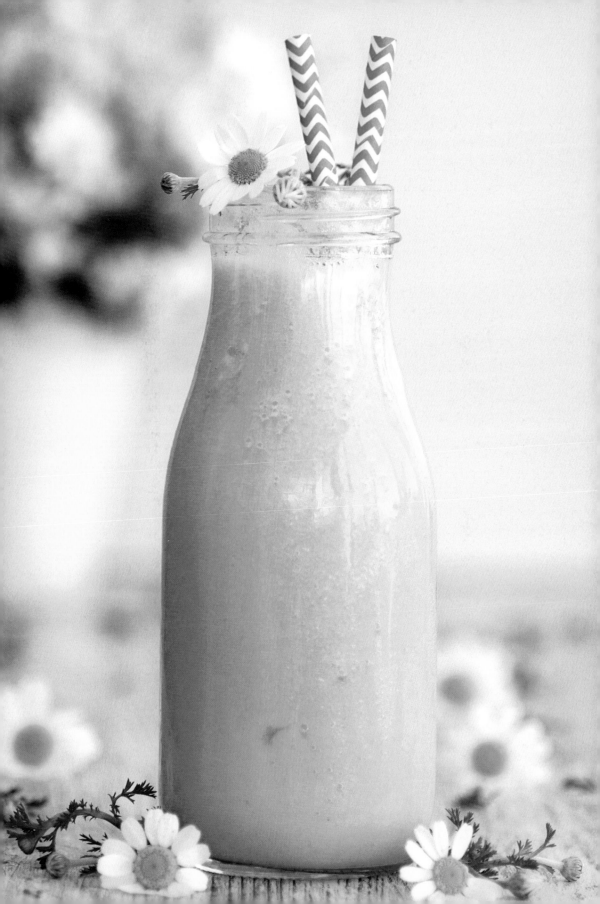

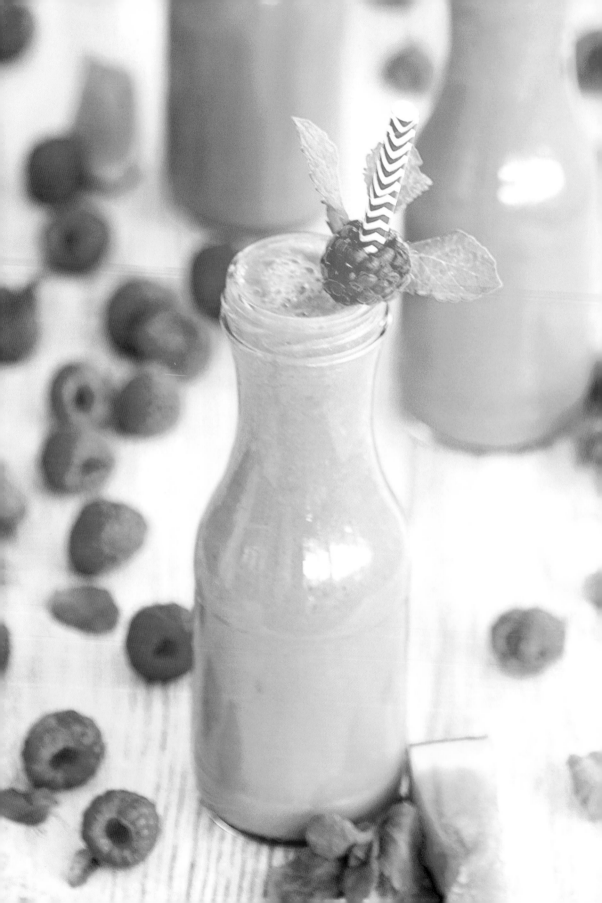

Pink Thunder

It is said that one single sea buckthorn berry contains as much vitamin C as a whole orange. However, the vitamin C content of sea buckthorn varies from 100 to 1,300 milligrams per 100 gram depending on the variety and degree of ripeness. Unusually for a plant, sea buckthorn contains vitamin B12, which is particularly important for vegetarians, but it also contains vitamins B1, B2, B3 (niacin), B6, B9 (folic acid), pantothenic acid, biotin, vitamin E, and vitamin K.

Sea buckthorn grows wild, but in recent years, commercial cultivation has become more widespread in the Nordic countries, Eastern Europe, Asia, the United States, and Canada. It is dioecious, i.e., it produces both male and female plants. A female plant produces berries after being pollinated by a male plant. Male plants sometimes produce berries too, but usually only small amounts. Sea buckthorn is wind-pollinated, so a good mixture of female and male plants is needed to ensure a supply of berries.

TIP
If your blender is less powerful, allow the raspberries to defrost a little before use.

MAKES 2 GLASSES

2–3 tsp sea buckthorn powder (or 1¾ oz / 50 g fresh or frozen berries)

7 oz / 200 g raspberries, frozen

7 oz / 200 g watermelon, cubed

1 cup / 250 ml kefir or yogurt, Greek-style

1–2 tsp honey

Blend everything into a smooth consistency.

Blueberry Heaven

Blueberries contain powerful antioxidants and are sometimes called superberries. They are good for the skin, eyesight, and night vision, and they counteract glaucoma. Blueberries are also said to be good for blood circulation in the legs and for combatting varicose veins, inflammation, blood clots, high blood pressure, and "bad" LDL cholesterol. Because they regulate blood sugar, blueberries are also considered beneficial to those with diabetes. Blueberries can also be helpful in the treatment of urinary tract infections and diarrhea.

Wild blueberries are particularly good for you as they have an abundance of flavonoids, carotene, vitamin C, vitamin B6, and magnesium.

MAKES 2 GLASSES

5½ oz / 150 g blueberries, wild, frozen

1½ cups / 350 ml Greek yogurt

1 tsp vanilla powder or extract

2 tsp raw honey

1 tsp bee pollen

2 tsp hemp seeds, shelled

ice

Blend all ingredients into a heavenly smoothie. If you are using fresh blueberries, blend in the ice at the end.

TIP
Greek yogurt is easy to make yourself and so much tastier—it is cheap, healthy, and simple. There is a recipe for home-made Greek yogurt on page 44.

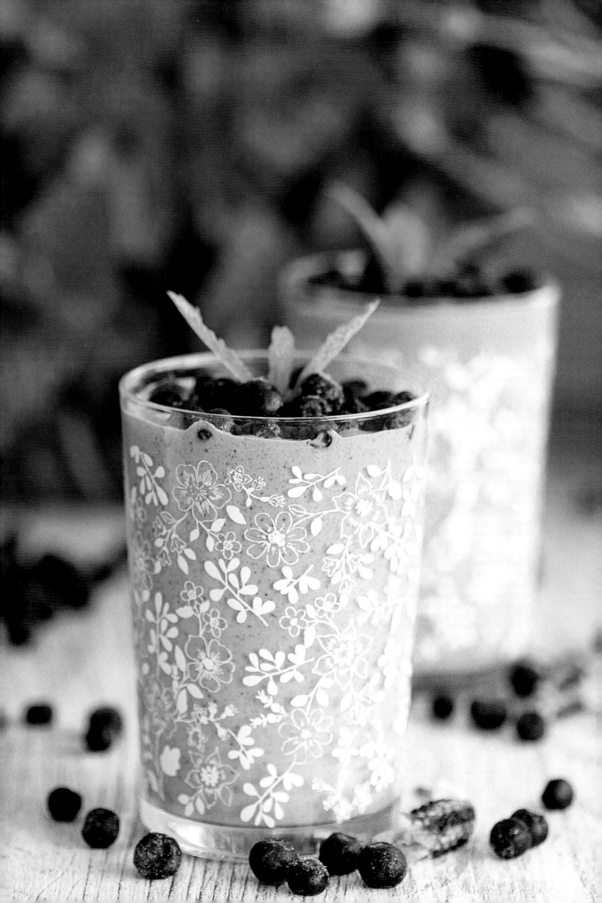

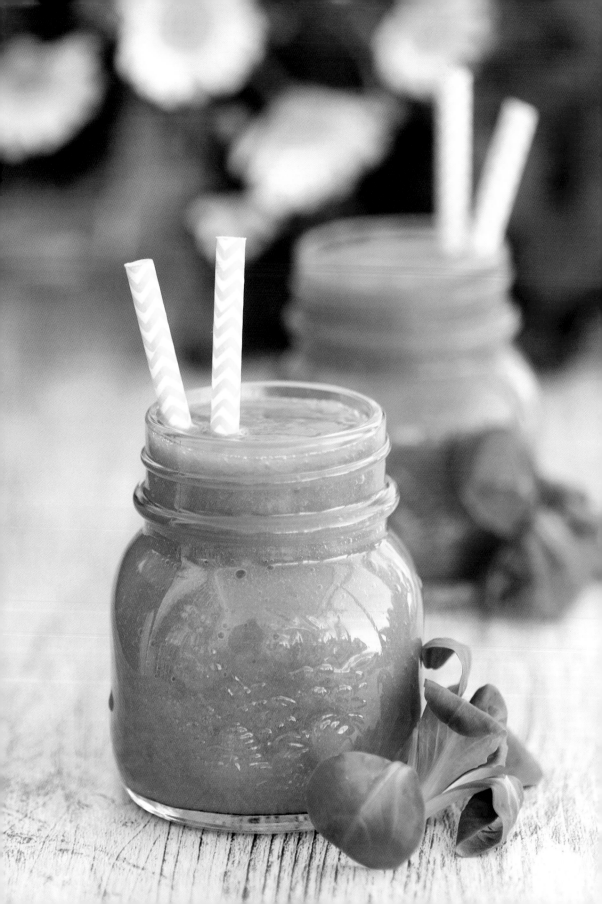

Rejuvenating Potion

Avocados are chock full of healthy fats that are said to prevent wrinkles and increase brain capacity. They have also long been considered an aphrodisiac. In addition to its possible stimulative effects and its healthy, monunsaturated fats, avocados also contain several nutrients that are beneficial for the blood, liver, heart, skin, and hair. Avocados contain large amounts of vitamin E, which makes the skin soft, supple, and healthy, and the hair extra shiny. It is also high in potassium, which helps to regulate blood pressure and is good for the muscles. Avocados also contain lots of fiber, folic acid, vitamins A, B, and C, and magnesium.

MAKES 2 GLASSES

2 avocados, pitted and peeled

2 oz / 60 g spinach

1 cup / 250 ml rejuvelac

⅔ cup / 150 ml apple juice, freshly pressed

1 banana

juice of 1 lime

Blend all the ingredients into a smooth consistency.

TIP
I like to blend or mash the avocado and use it as a face mask once or twice a week, and also as a mask for the whole body or the hair. The only downside is that you have to clean up the shower a bit afterwards, but because the avocado makes your skin and hair look so good, I feel it is worth it.

Wild Flowerberry

Bee pollen, also called bee pollen granules, is a fantastic supplement that is packed with nourishment. Bee pollen provides virtually all the nutrients the body needs to maintain and build up good health. It contains up to 200 bioactive substances and provides more concentrated nourishment than fruit and vegetables. Amongst its contents are 22 different amino acids, antioxidants such as bioflavonoids and polyphenols, 27 minerals, and 16 vitamins.

Bee pollen is known for strengthening the immune system, enhancing concentration and memory, increasing sexual desire and fertility, curbing the appetite, speeding up the metabolism, and providing an energy boost.

Bee pollen grains vary in color and taste because bees collect pollen from different flowers, which affects the taste and smell, and vegetation changes with the season. But it has a floral taste whatever the time of year.

Another exciting thing about pollen is that it may be able to combat hay fever. If you take pollen from a local source for a few weeks before flowers come into bloom in the spring, it can relieve allergy problems and, in some cases, cure them altogether.

MAKES 2 GLASSES

1 cup / 250 ml chamomile tea, cooled

7 oz / 200 g wild strawberries

2 pears, cored

1 cup / 250 ml kombucha

2 tsp raw honey

1 tsp bee pollen

ice

Make the tea and cool. Blend all the ingredients into a smooth consistency. For a colder smoothie, add some ice at the end.

IS IT SAFE?

Bee pollen is safe for most people, but if you are allergic to pollen you should be careful. Start by doing the tongue test—put a very small amount of bee pollen on your tongue to see if it irritates the throat or sinuses. If nothing happens, it should be fine for you to use bee pollen and enjoy all the health benefits it brings.

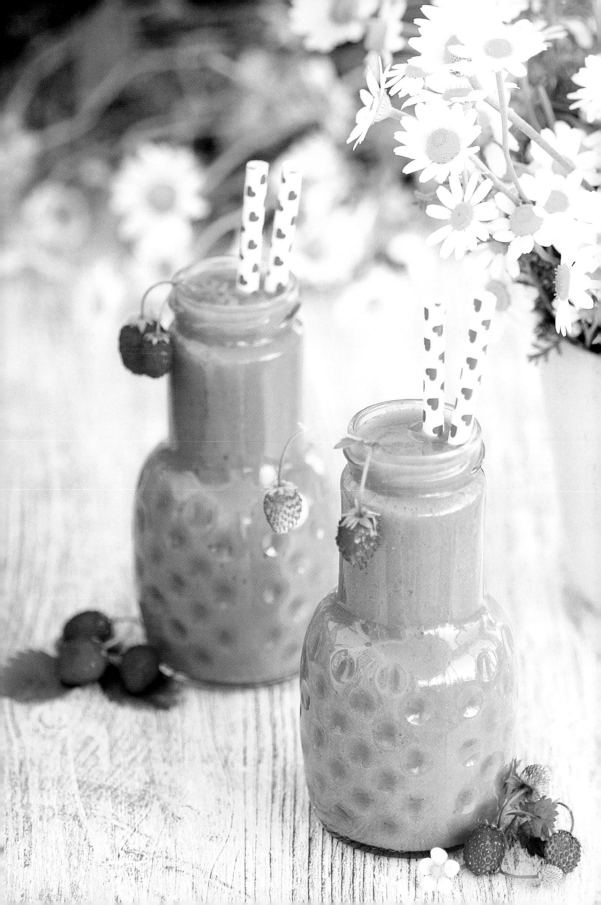

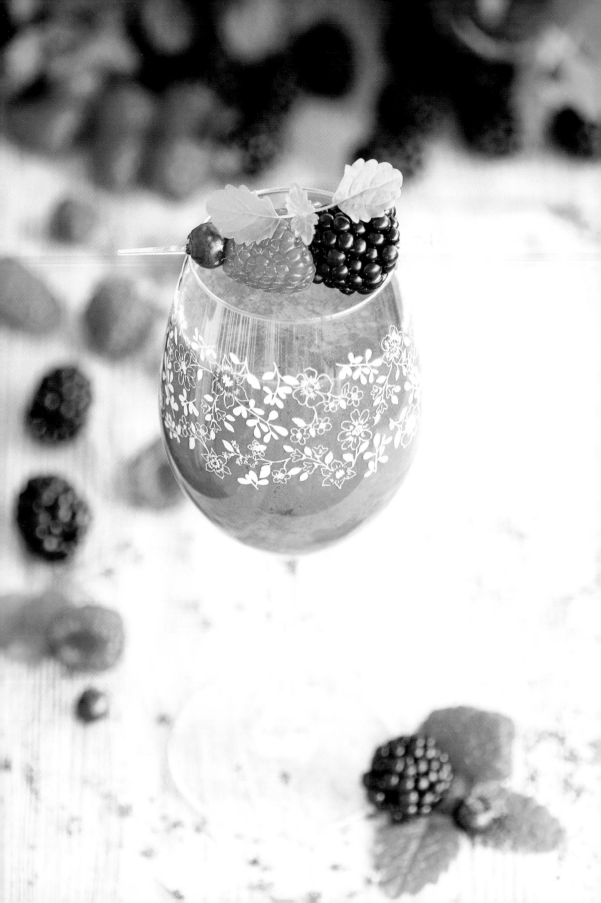

Berrybucha

Redcurrants contain large amounts of vitamins C and K, and potassium, and a lot of fiber. Currants are normally grown in gardens, but there is a wild subspecies of currant that grows freely where I live—you can go out into the forest and pick some. And you can actually make good wine from currants, both wild and cultivated ones. It is always best to use the fruit when in season and freeze when large quantities are available.

MAKES 2 GLASSES

5½ oz / 150 g redcurrants, frozen

1¾ oz / 50 g raspberries, frozen

1¾ oz / 50 g blackberries, frozen

1¾ oz / 50 g blackcurrants, frozen

1 banana

1⅔ cups / 400 ml kombucha

1–2 Medjool dates, pitted

TIP
If your blender is less powerful, allow the berries to defrost a little before use. You can use any combination of berries, and, if you want sweetness but do not wish to use dates, banana or pineapple will enhance the flavor.

Tropical Wild Strawberry

Wild or woodland strawberries (*fragaria vesca*) have a wonderful smell, taste delightful, and are often associated with sunny days spent in the forest as a child—memories of red, sun-ripened berries threaded onto endless blades of grass. Wild strawberries are my beloved three-year-old daughter's favorite berry. She picks them for herself in our garden—where they have replaced all the flowers.

Wild strawberries are very easy to grow and will produce fruit from early spring right up until the frosts arrive. There are also other types of wild strawberry—*fragaria moschata* and *fragaria viridis*—that grow wild and are even more flavorsome than home-grown varieties.

MAKES 2 GLASSES

7 oz / 200 g wild strawberries
(or regular strawberries)

1¾ oz / 50 g cloudberries

5½ oz / 150 g pineapple, frozen

1⅔ cups / 400 ml water kefir

Blend all the ingredients into a heavenly smoothie.

TIP
If wild strawberries are hard to find, replace with regular strawberries and add 1¾ oz or 50 grams of cloudberries. The cloudberries further enhance the delicious flavor of the wild strawberries.

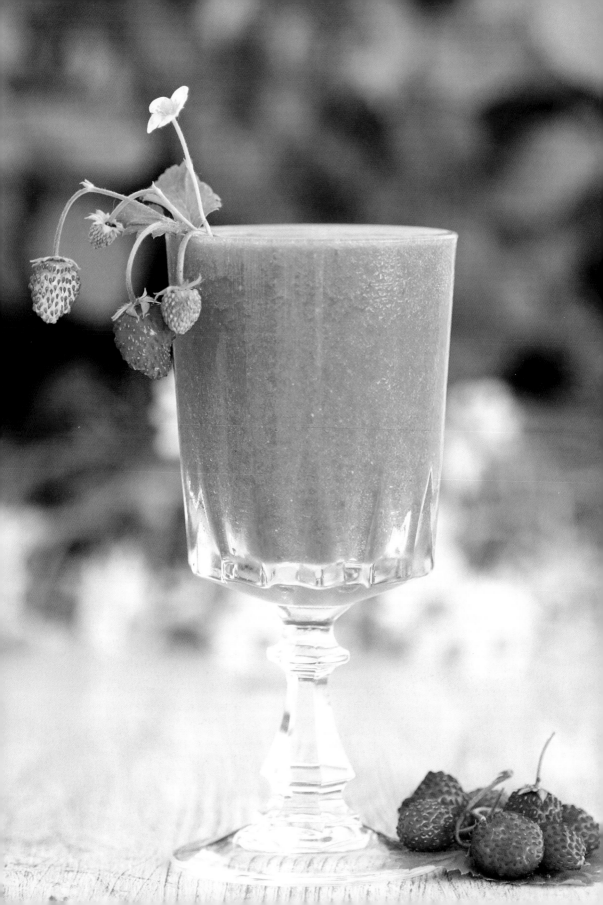

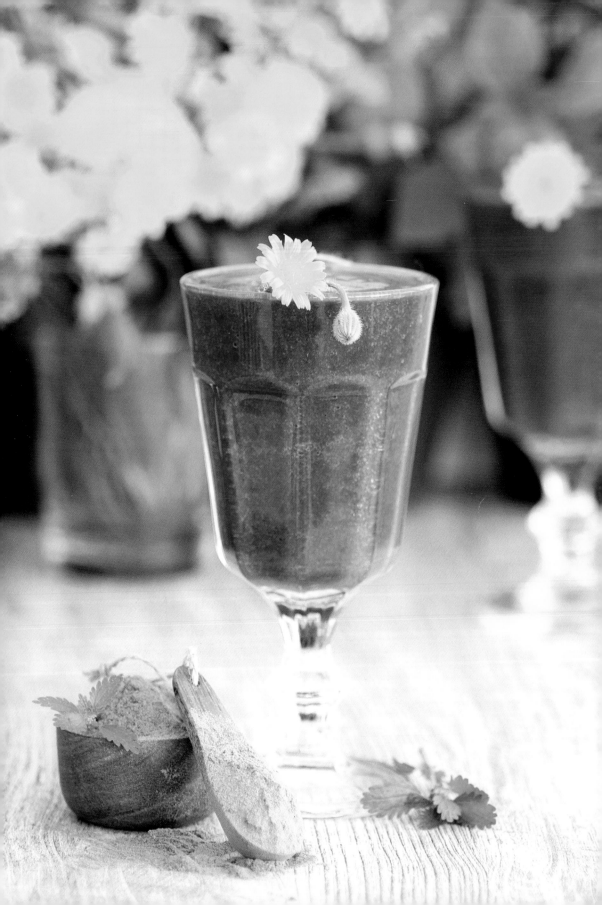

Probiotic Weed

Ground elder (*Aegopodium podagraria*) is one of our commonest weeds , but is actually edible and really good for you. Like other green-leaved vegetables, ground elder is full of vitamins and minerals. It can be eaten hot or cold, in smoothies, soups, pies, salads, pesto, or in vegetarian patties.

I am always pleased to see the first shoots of ground elder appear each year. It means I will soon be able to enjoy one of my most favorite vegetables. Ground elder is not in fact a weed, it is a domesticated vegetable that has run wild, having previously been cultivated by gardeners such as monks and nuns. If you have ground elder in your garden—congratulations. You will never need to buy spinach again.

MAKES 2 GLASSES

1 cup / 250 ml dandelion tea

1 cup / 250 ml kombucha or water kefir

2 oz / 60 g ground elder, crisp leaves

1 tsp nettle powder or a handful of fresh leaves (soaked for at least 30 minutes)

2 apples, cored

1–2 Medjool dates, pitted

Blend all the ingredients into a delicious, green health boost.

NOTE
Do not harvest ground elder without identifying the plant with the help of a good flower book. Never eat a plant if you are not certain of its identity.

Abbreviations and Quantities

1 oz = 1 ounce = 28 grams
1 lb = 1 pound = 16 ounces 1
1 cup = approx. 5–8 ounces* (see below)
1 cup = 8 fl uid ounces = 250 milliliters (liquids)
2 cups = 1 pint (liquids) = 15 milliliters (liquids)
8 pints = 4 quarts = 1 gallon (liquids)
1 g = 1 gram = 1/1000 kilogram = 5 ml (liquids)
1 kg = 1 kilogram = 1000 grams = 2¼ lb
1 l = 1 liter = 1000 milliliters (ml) = 1 quart
125 milliliters (ml) = approx. 8 tablespoons = ½ cup
1 tbsp = 1 level tablespoon = 15–20 g* (depending on density) = 15 milliliters (liquids)
1 tsp = 1 level teaspoon = 3–5 g * (depending on density) = 5 ml (liquids)

*The weight of dry ingredients varies significantly depending on the density factor, e.g. 1 cup of flour weighs less than 1 cup of butter. Quantities in ingredients have been rounded up or down for convenience, where appropriate. Metric conversions may therefore not correspond exactly.
It is important to use either American or metric measurements within a recipe.

WARNING!

Never shake fermented drinks in their bottles and do not swirl the liquid around before you open it, especially if it is flavored, as fermentation will still be in progress. The drinks are carbonated, and you need to handle them with the same care as you would champagne or any other carbonated drink. Any glass bottles you use *must* be pressure-resistant, or you can use BPA PET bottles approved for food use. Both must have a tight-fitting stopper. Other types of bottle may explode. As a precaution, store the bottles in a closed box such as a picnic coolbox, so that if the bottles do explode, any damage or cleaning required will be minimal.

You should release the pressure from time to time, preferably wrapping a clean towel around the opening while you open the bottle extremely carefully, a little at a time. If you are using a flavoring that ferments, use only a little (5–10%) as, particularly with very sweet fruit, it will produce a lot of gas and the contents might spurt out as you open the bottle before you have had a chance to taste it. I know—I have tried it.

The more fruit you use, the greater the risk of having to spend hours cleaning.

The information and recipes in this book have been compiled with the utmost care and provided to the best of our knowledge and belief, and from our own experience. However, neither the publisher, nor the author nor the translator shall accept liability for any misadventure or harm resulting directly or indirectly from the information given in this book. This disclaimer applies in particular to the use and consumption of untreated raw milk and/or raw milk products, which the author and publisher strongly advise against due to the associated health risks. When in doubt, always consult your GP.

Please note that bee pollen can be dangerous to those with allergies to bees, their products or other seasonal allergies.

It is essential to always take the necessary precautions and keep everything clean while working with fermented drinks.

© Eliq Maranik and Stevali Production

Text and photos: Eliq Maranik
Photos of Eliq: Anna Enström Shine Photography
Art Director: Eliq Maranik and Liis Karu
Design: Liis Karu
Editor: Eva Stjerne, Ord & Form

© for the English edition: h.f.ullmann publishing GmbH

Translation from Swedish:
Edwina Simpson, in association with
First Edition Translations Ltd, Cambridge, UK.

Overall responsibility for production: h.f.ullmann publishing GmbH, Potsdam, Germany

Printed in Slovenia, 2017

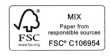

MIX
Paper from responsible sources
FSC® C106954

ISBN 978-3-8480-1110-0

10 9 8 7 6 5 4 3 2 1
X IX VIII VII VI IV III II I

www.ullmannmedien.com
info@ullmannmedien.com
facebook.com/ullmannmedien
twitter.com/ullmann_int